DOCTORS TO BE

DOCTORS
TO BE

Susan Spindler

BBC Books

To David, Dong, Ese, Fey, Jane, John, Mark, Nick, Sarah
and Will, who endured the cameras and the questions with
patience and fortitude.

Picture Credits

Princess Diana outside Lindo Wing, Alan Davidson/Camera Press;
Historical pictures, anatomy class and operating theatre photos,
courtesy St Mary's Hospital Medical School, with special thanks
to Kevin Brown, Archivist and Librarian; Musical Revue photo
courtesy Clare Nettleton; Rugby Club photo courtesy Neal Hunt.
All other photos © BBC & Radio Times (photographers Jeremy
Grayson and David Edwards).

ISBN 0 563 36095 X

First published in hardback by BBC Books,
a division of BBC Enterprises Limited,
Woodlands, 80 Wood Lane, London W12 0TT

Set in $11\frac{1}{2}$/14pt Baskerville Roman, by Butler and Tanner Ltd, Frome, Somerset
Jacket printed by Lawrence Allen Ltd, Weston-super-Mare
Printed and bound by Butler and Tanner Ltd, Frome, Somerset

CONTENTS

ACKNOWLEDGEMENTS

My greatest debt is to the ten doctors-to-be who appear in both the book and the television series: their commitment, enthusiasm and good humour have been remarkable during eight years of work on the series. I am also grateful to all the staff of St Mary's Hospital and Medical School who have supported the project. In particular, without the encouragement and assistance of the Dean, Peter Richards, who was ready to see his own establishment assessed and criticised in order to create an accurate record of an era of medical training, the series could not have been made, nor this book written.

At St Mary's I also received considerable help from the archivist Kevin Brown, the deputy registrar Walter Umpleby and staff at the medical school library. Gill Arscott and Susan English answered endless enquiries with patience and efficiency.

Hundreds of patients at St Mary's and the other hospitals where our students were taught agreed to take part in filming and their experiences are reflected in this book. Many of them were ill, anxious and in pain and a few knew that they had only a short time to live: I am particularly grateful for their generosity and interest in the project. Similarly, nursing and medical staff on the wards were always helpful and accommodating, even at times when they were extremely hard-pressed.

Thanks are due to all those at the BBC whose wisdom, experience and dedication to the series have helped me immeasurably:

in particular Edward Briffa, the series producer and mainstay of the project, who shared many insights, gave continuous technical aid and never lost his temper; Robin Brightwell, the series editor; and Valerie Patten, who brought enthusiasm and efficiency to the final stages of writing and checking and prepared the manuscript immaculately. All three read the text and made invaluable suggestions.

The original idea for the television series came from Jon Palfreman. Michael Haynes, Dave Gray, Tim Watts, Martin Cooper, Colin Goudie, Mike Flynn, Alison Lewis, Andrew Metcalf, Alex McLeod, Pat Greenland, Fiona Holmes, Judith Bunting, Clare O'Donovan, Suzan Walker, John Lilley, Jane Evans, Anne Edwards and Anne Cafferky all contributed substantially to the programmes between 1985 and 1992.

Isobel Allan, Elizabeth Shore and Beulah Bewley made time to see me to discuss undergraduate and postgraduate medical education and I am indebted to them for information and analysis. Caroline van den Brul and Vanessa Harvey-Samuel read the manuscript and made many useful comments. Debbie Shephard sacrificed some of her privacy for the sake of a truer picture of the house officer year.

At home a succession of splendid au pairs – Ute Meier, Cordula Krauss-Laib, Cosima Wrassman and Katja Promess – were the pillars of my support. A special tribute is due to my parents and particularly to my husband Peter and our children Toby, Matthew and Imogen, who suffered long periods of absence while I grappled with recalcitrant word processors. To their relief that the book is finished, I add my heartfelt thanks.

SS

INTRODUCTION

In 1983, the BBC decided to make a series about the training of doctors, following a group of medical students from the moment they applied to medical school until they qualified – and beyond, as they pursued their careers.

The first task was to approach a few medical schools to see if any was willing to play host to a television crew for a minimum of six years. Several schools were contacted and eventually St Mary's in Paddington, west London, emerged as favourite. The Dean of St Mary's, Professor Peter Richards, was enthusiastic about the idea. 'When I was first approached I could foresee a number of potential problems, and knew that there was a substantial risk involved, but I felt that medical education was a legitimate subject for public interest and someone, somewhere had the responsibility of laying the system open to examination. A few of my colleagues on the Academic Board were completely hostile to the idea, but we had a discussion, and in the end the adventurous ones won.'

The combination of unfettered access to lectures, seminars, outpatient clinics and wards, and a Dean who believed in the project made St Mary's the obvious choice. The BBC producers promised that filming would be 'fly on the wall' – that is, the cameras would record events as they occurred, rather than setting up action in advance and filming repeated 'takes' of the same scene, as so often happens in documentary film making – and that the BBC team would interfere as little as possible with the normal working of the hospital and medical school.

St Mary's placed few restrictions on the BBC. The crews could film anywhere within the hospital and medical school – with the proviso that all patients, students and teaching staff must be happy to participate. There were two important exceptions which were outside the control of the medical school: dissection of cadavers in the anatomy department, which was controlled by the Home Office, and examinations, which were organised by London University, even though they took place on St Mary's premises. A clause in the contract stipulated that the medical school could request the removal of any material which it thought might damage the career of a particular student.

Filming began in November 1984, during the annual admissions interviews: 419 applicants were called for interview and 100 of the interviews were filmed (interviewees had been warned about the presence of cameras in advance by letter, and given the opportunity to opt out). The following autumn, when the successful candidates arrived at St Mary's to begin their medical careers, the whole year was asked if it wished to be involved in the making of the programmes and responded positively.

Then came the selection of our doctors in the making: ten students who would agree to long-term television coverage. The choice was difficult; there were diverse and interesting characters among the 1985 intake, but those selected needed to be outgoing, resilient and long-suffering if they were to cope with the presence of cameras throughout their student years, not only during periods of initiation, enjoyment and celebration, but also in times of exhaustion, failure and uncertainty. In the event ten were chosen: Dong Ching Chiu, David Copping, Mark George, Sarah Holdsworth, Nick Hollings, William Liddell, Jane Morris, Ese Oshevire, Fey Probst and John Shephard.

The series aimed to give a picture of their life at medical school in eight programmes which would cover seven years. The narrative threads of the series were inextricably entangled in the lives of our ten students. We tried to imagine how they might fare – though many of our hunches turned out to be wrong!

We wondered what would happen to them: would they pass or

fail? Would they like medicine, or hate it and drop out of medical school? How many of them would end up practising as doctors? How would their attitudes and values change during those seven critical years in their development? Each of the students was filmed regularly. In the end, more than three hundred hours of material were recorded.

'There was a lot of suspicion during the first two years,' recalled the Dean, 'followed by a grudging acceptance of the cameras. But now practically everyone is pleased and proud to be associated with the project, and there is a general feeling that the series has captured the flavour of the educational experience, including its crises and moments of truth. The series shows an educational process which has changed little for a century and which has now been captured before it disappears.'

1

TRIAL BY INTERVIEW

Nick Hollings sat in the beige-brown medical school corridor, waiting for his name to be called. A curly-haired, eighteen-year-old public school cherub in a sports jacket, he looked confident, but he knew that the next few minutes might determine the course of his whole life.

It was the autumn of 1984, a season now fixed in the public memory by the IRA bombing of the Conservative Party conference at Brighton. Nick was one of almost two and a half thousand people who had applied for a seat in the corridor, making St Mary's the second most popular medical school in the country. Interviews had been offered to 419 candidates – those with the best exam results and school reports, whose application forms also revealed wide interests and enthusiasms.

Today's aspiring doctors are allowed to apply to five medical schools, without ranking them, but in 1984, applicants had to list their five schools in order of preference. The order they chose was a significant feature of the admissions procedure. Oxford and Cambridge, for example, were known to discard applications from candidates who did not place them first.

Nick Hollings, the son of a dentist and a teacher, who had just left Shrewsbury School with three good A levels, had every reason to feel confident of a place somewhere. He had put St Mary's bottom of his list – a fact, as he well knew, that would not necessarily endear him to the interview panel.

More than a quarter of British medical schools select the doctors of the future simply by picking out the most impressive forms. But St Mary's sets great store by the interview and tries to see as many applicants as possible. Most interviewees are still at school and have not yet sat their A levels. All the interviewers are doctors or academics, however, and the many pressures on their time restrict the average length of an interview to fifteen minutes.

Many of the candidates visiting St Mary's in 1984 had never been interviewed for a university place; most of them were seventeen, and, unlike Nick, had not yet taken their A levels. They knew that this might be their only chance to embark on a medical training: everything hung on the next ten or fifteen minutes. Like Nick Hollings, most candidates came by train, walking the few hundred metres from Paddington Station up Praed Street, a noisy cosmopolitan introduction to the inner city, then sharp left through wrought iron gates and into Norfolk Place, a small space dominated by the Victorian hospital on one side and the 1930s buildings of the medical school on the other. Inside, candidates huddled nervously in the ground floor corridors, strangers attempting brittle conversation, until one of the chairmen emerged to claim another victim.

Each candidate faced a panel of three: a practising doctor, a scientist and a chairman. In 1984 the role of chairman was shared between four people: the Dean of St Mary's, Professor Peter Richards; Dr George Tait, the Senior Pre-Clinical Tutor; Professor John Sirs, a biophysicist; and the Professor of Anatomy, Aidan Breathnach. The presence of one of these senior members of the medical school throughout the interview season was designed to give consistency to the interview process.

Nick Hollings' chairman was the Dean, a small, thin man in his mid-fifties with the half-moon spectacles, cerebral intensity and eloquence of an old-style Oxbridge don. The son of a GP, he had trained in medicine at Cambridge and at St George's Hospital Medical School in London where he managed to win academic prizes as well as playing university standard hockey and teaching himself Swedish. He was appointed Dean in 1979 and now ran a medical school that employed more than 650 staff and had an annual budget of £18 million. Although he had a punishing administrative routine of meetings and paperwork, Peter Richards continued to look after patients and teach medical students. Despite his steely politeness towards candidates and ready smile, he could be a cunning interviewer, stealthily encouraging his guests into admissions of ignorance or displays of bombast, then puncturing their composure with a carefully-honed rejoinder.

Mr Hollings, as the Dean called him, was shown to 'the hot seat' – a chair placed at one end of a long table, in a bland, featureless room. As well as the Dean he faced Dr Stuart Montgomery, a consultant psychiatrist, and Mrs Jane Wadsworth, a statistician. Dr Montgomery fired a daunting opening question: 'What direction do you think medicine will be going in during the next twenty years?' But Nick took it well. 'I think recombinant DNA and genetic engineering is obviously an exploding field in science,' he began, launching into an impressive display of familiarity with current developments in molecular biology. This seemed to encourage the panel to move into a higher gear. Asked what changes he would advise the minister of health to make in the NHS he replied, 'Crumbs!' But he quickly went on to suggest the use of private medical insurance to fund old people's homes, while cleverly acknowledging that there could be some attendant problems. He was making the best use he could of his fifteen minutes.

He kept his end up well, never appeared rattled and even succeeded in imposing his own agenda on the interview. He emerged as a right winger: laissez-faire on smoking, pessimistic about the chances of solving the medical problems of the third world, and an enthusiast for private medicine. Nick was thanked and shown out, and the panel sat in silence for a few minutes, writing notes.

St Mary's has devised its own system for grading candidates: A, make an offer; B1, make an offer, competition permitting, otherwise leave on the waiting list; B2, place on waiting list, pending A level results; and C, reject. The Dean was evidently impressed with Nick – he gave him an A. But Dr Montgomery felt he detected naivety and arrogance and consequently gave him a B1. So did Mrs Wadsworth, though she had liked him very much. In the subsequent discussion the Dean won the day and the panel decided to make Nick an unconditional offer. Privately, they doubted whether he would accept it.

In fact, Nick was rejected by his first choice, Cambridge, and liked St Mary's so much that he turned down places at Manchester and Bristol in order to accept the offer there.

The only immediately discernible similarity between Nick Hollings and Ese Oshevire was that both had placed Cambridge top of their lists of medical schools. Ese was born in Sheffield in 1966 to a Nigerian couple. Both her parents worked full-time and they needed to find a temporary foster home for the new baby. Mrs Marina White, a Chesterfield miner's wife, noticed the advertisement they had placed in a Sheffield evening paper and remarked to her four sons that it was a shame that no one had taken in the little baby. 'You're no better,' scolded her eldest son. 'We've got room, why don't we have her here?' Mrs White decided that he was right, and she and her husband volunteered to foster Ese, then aged two months.

Ese was brought up as one of the family, although she never lost contact with her Nigerian parents, two sisters and brother. Marina White was Mam and her real mother was Mum. At the age of seven her father took her to Nigeria to live with her family but after a year she chose to return, homesick for Derbyshire and her foster family. She attended a state primary school and St Helena's Secondary High School, a girls' comprehensive in Chesterfield. There were no doctors in her family and she had very little idea what a career in medicine would be like. St Mary's was her fourth choice.

The interview went well; Ese, a bubbly, extrovert girl with a broad Derbyshire accent, felt the panel were intrigued by her numerous interests. She was an outstanding athlete and netball player who did modern dance and judo as well as being deputy head girl at school. 'It was a nice interview, very different from Cambridge, where they asked very difficult questions which I didn't understand.'

Cambridge turned her down but St Mary's gave Ese its standard offer – a B and two Cs at A Level – and although she had placed it fourth on her application form, she was so impressed with the school that she accepted. 'It was small and very friendly,' said Ese. 'People I met when I toured the medical school seemed to welcome me with open arms.' She secured her place with A, B and C grades in her science A levels.

'I think I was a sort of experiment for the medical school: Nigerian, social class 5 and from the north of England. They were probably surprised to find someone who was black, with a foster-father who was a miner, who came from a little school in Chesterfield and yet had all these achievements – especially when there were all these people from public schools turning up in suits. They must have thought: "Let's give her a chance!" ' The Dean was keen on outside interests: 'Doing anything well – playing sport or music, collecting butterflies, writing articles – requires an enormous amount of application and perseverance, and I think that can be moved sideways and applied to medicine.'

The interviewers were also trying to assess how active a candidate was likely to be in the social and cultural life of St Mary's. 'London medical schools have a long tradition of accepting academically able students on the basis of their wider interests, abilities and attitudes, not on A level grades alone,' explained the Dean. 'This policy makes for a widely talented, active student community. We look for people with some evidence of originality and broad interests who have made a contribution to their own school and local community and who we feel will also make a contribution here.'

Jane Morris was typical of the kind of bright all-rounder that St Mary's was trying to attract. The daughter of a company director, she was formidably well-qualified, with eleven grade As at O level, a glowing testimonial from her school – Olchfa Comprehensive near Swansea, which predicted similar success at A level – and a huge range of outside interests. Drama was her greatest love. St Mary's traditionally draws a significant proportion of its intake from south Wales, and several old pupils from Jane's school were among the current students; she knew the college had a strong theatrical tradition.

It was Jane's first interview, but despite her nervousness, she appeared poised and confident. A pretty, vivacious girl with a black bob, she had the middle-aged gentlemen of the panel eating out of her hand within minutes of entering the interview room. She spoke with shining eyes of a recent 'character building' expedition in the Brecon Beacons, undertaken as part of her Duke of Edinburgh Award scheme, and of her lifelong determination to study medicine. 'For the past three years I have worked at my local hospital every Sunday morning, so I know what medicine entails.' She also confessed to reading a lot of literature – 'especially Shakespeare'.

All three members of the panel awarded Jane an A and felt that she should be put forward as a scholarship candidate. 'She comes from a comprehensive school and she's done extraordinarily well,' commented one interviewer. 'She was an excellent, thoughtful, mature candidate, and also very engaging.' Because they were so keen to tempt her, St Mary's made Jane a very low offer: three Cs. And although it had been her third choice, Jane was so impressed by her visit to the school that she accepted the offer. She got two As and a B in her A levels.

One of the standard questions in the interviews was: 'Why do you want to study medicine?' This was where a layman might have expected a sense of vocation to emerge, but few candidates would have put it as strongly as that. Most of them simply wanted to help people, and saw medicine as a job that combined this with the study of science. Some, like David Copping, a pre-A level candidate from High Wycombe, had experienced ill health and decided to aim for medicine after seeing a doctor at work. 'As a young child, I wanted to be a pilot,' recalled David, 'but then I got hay fever and asthma and so that went out of the window. When I was about thirteen, I became very ill with asthma while we were on holiday and a doctor friend of my parents treated me and tried out lots of different drugs until eventually I got better – it struck me as a very satisfying thing to do. At first people told me I didn't have the brains for it. My O levels weren't brilliant, but I suppose I was a late developer and I improved in the sixth form.'

David was a pupil at Wycombe Royal Grammar School, an intensely academic state school which sent many boys to medical school every year. He applied to five London medical schools because they had a reputation for asking for lower A level grades than schools in other parts of Britain. St Mary's was David's first choice. He was shown round by a family friend who was a junior doctor. He liked the small scale and friendly atmosphere.

David also felt that his father's job as a vicar had given him an insight into what life would be like as a doctor. 'Living in a vicarage is a good training for medicine because it's like a social centre and it teaches you to get on with all sorts of people. As a small child I would come downstairs in my pyjamas at night and find my father speaking to a couple he was about to marry. Drunks occasionally turned up on the doorstep, and people would ring up in floods of tears and sometimes I ended up speaking to them because my parents were out. It's useful when you apply for medical school, because the admissions system is biased in favour of people who have developed social skills early and interview well. Some people haven't got them by the time they apply, because they've led very sheltered lives.'

David's interview was rather undemanding, amounting to little more than a recital of his interests and voluntary activities. He came over well and seemed relaxed and self-possessed. The panel asked questions about his work with handicapped children and his amateur beer making, but didn't probe him much. Their interest in him seemed to be whetted by his disclosure that he had also been invited to interviews at King's College Hospital and the Royal Free. After the interview the chairman, Dr Tait, summed up: 'A very sound young man.'

David was offered a place at St Mary's conditional on getting a B and two Cs at A level, and he accepted the offer. In the event he passed with two As and a C.

There is a widespread belief that medical school selection is biased in favour of the children of doctors. The Dean denies it. St Mary's, like most medical schools, automatically interviews the children of its graduates out of courtesy (candidates are required to state the parents' occupations on their application forms), but only eighteen per cent of both its applicants and its entrants are doctors' children, and very few of them have parents who attended St Mary's. Professor Richards emphasises that a central aim of the selection process is to achieve as diverse a mix of students as possible. 'We try very hard to take a wide cross-section of people, because we are trying to construct a community in which medical students will learn humanely, energetically and happily. We try to take as many good northerners as we can get, because I think there is a tendency to have a north-south divide in medical schools.'

Sarah Holdsworth, aged seventeen and a pre-A level candidate, was no doubt perceived as a 'good northerner' by her interview panel of southerners, headed by the Dean himself. Dressed with sober smartness in a white high-necked blouse, plaid skirt and dark blue jacket, Sarah saw her interview at St Mary's (her fourth choice) as a dry run for Nottingham University, which she had placed top of her list. Her background was not medical: her father read engineering at university and now held a senior position in local government, and her mother was a housewife who had travelled with her to Paddington from their home near Wigan, partly to keep her company and partly because she was nervous about Sarah visiting London alone. Wholesome, earnest, open-faced and utterly straightforward, Sarah had decided to take the advice of doctor friends who told her, 'Just be yourself and be confident.'

The interviewers tended to begin with a question about the candidate's interests in order to relax tensions and get him or her used to the environment. It was generally a successful ploy – although those who tried to pass off vague interests as all-consuming passions on their application forms risked falling at this first hurdle. Sarah soon embarked on a bracing recitation of her favourite sports, sailing, lacrosse and swimming. She played the organ, violin and piano, and worked for a Duke of Edinburgh Award. She was a venture scout and 'middle school dining room prefect' at Bolton School, a local independent school.

Asked where she would really like to go to medical school, Sarah was forthright. 'Obviously, I'd like to go to Nottingham most. It's only two hours from home on the train. I know someone who's already there and she loves it. And they play lacrosse.' She explained that she had always wanted to do medicine. 'It's a challenge, because it is a difficult job and I think you probably get a lot of job satisfaction. I work best under pressure and like working with people. The chances of getting a job at the end of training are good – and I suppose the wages are good.' The Dean smiled into his paperwork before beginning his questions. Why did people become tramps? Sarah was flummoxed; she suggested despair, unemployment and poverty. The Dean was looking for alcoholism.

After Sarah had left the room, still puzzling over the tramp question, the interviewers compared notes. The Dean rated her as an A candidate, consultant geriatrician Dr Angela Middleton thought her a B1 and Dr Sheila Wilson gave her a B2 'simply because I don't think she'll come here'. 'Neither do I,' replied the Dean, 'but I think she'd be very good and we lose nothing by giving her an offer, except a postage stamp.' He took the view that 'if we would like to have somebody here, we make them an offer and hope that during the course of the day they change their mind, which happens a lot.'

It happened to Sarah. She loved St Mary's and her mother, who had spent the day in the medical school waiting for her, liked the atmosphere and felt that, after all, she would not mind Sarah coming to London to study. Sarah rejected Nottingham and accepted the St Mary's offer of a B and two Cs. She managed it comfortably, passing with A, B and C grades.

St Mary's students put a lot of effort into giving candidates who attend for interview a tempting glimpse of what the medical school had to offer. Candidates were taken on a tour of the place by a current student and shown the dissecting room, lecture theatres and labs, student bar and swimming pool. They were also taken on to the wards and introduced to doctors, nurses and other medical students. The tour leader also explained the structure of the course and described the clubs and societies which provided Mary's students with a famously hectic social life. Most candidates came away with a very favourable impression.

The interview tour played a critical part in shaping the medical career of seventeen-year-old Mark George, who travelled to St Mary's from Hertfordshire where he was a day boy at St Alban's School. Mark had applied to five London medical schools. 'I knew that I wanted to work in London afterwards, so I thought it would be an advantage to go to a London teaching hospital. I had already visited Bart's and Charing Cross, so I put them first and second and St Mary's, which I hadn't seen, third. But when I visited Mary's for my interview, I was very taken with it. The friendly atmosphere, good facilities and accommodation all appealed to me and by the end of the day there I badly wanted to get an offer.'

Mark was a relaxed, sociable boy with an insouciant grin, who had always done well at school. He played the piano and the trumpet and was keen on sport, especially hockey. He had wanted to be a doctor since going into hospital at the age of nine to have his adenoids removed. There was no medical tradition in his family – his father was a marketing manager and his mother a secretary – but he told his parents his ambition, they gave him a book called *The Human Body*, and he had never looked back.

He chose his A level subjects – Maths, Physics and Chemistry – with medicine in mind. His mother arranged for him to spend three weeks at the local district hospital where he watched a variety of operations and was confirmed in his choice of career. His motives for entering medicine echoed his childhood enthusiasm: 'I wanted to learn more about science and more about how the body works. Money and status weren't considerations at all. I just wanted a job I would really enjoy.'

Mark's interview took place in November 1984. 'It was my first interview for medical school and I was quite nervous. When I first arrived at Paddington, I couldn't find my way out of the station and got into a bit of a panic. I eventually managed to find the right building just in time for my interview. They asked me about doctors and the nuclear arms race and the issue of confidentiality of patients' notes. When I came out I didn't have a clue how it had gone. The next day, I had an interview at Charing Cross and they sent me an offer the following day, but I sat on it for a while, hoping I would hear from Mary's. They finally sent me an offer of a B and two Cs and I was absolutely over the moon. I accepted immediately.'

At five years, medicine is one of the longest university courses in

Britain and the most expensive – it costs the country more than £150 000 to train a doctor (1991 values). Most medical students at St Mary's received local authority grants, but there were a few students there who received no financial help with their studies: foreign students paid £50 000 in tuition fees (1991 values) for the five-year course. Competition was particularly fierce among these students: in 1984 there were 1723 applicants for the 213 places available to them in British medical schools. St Mary's was allowed to take up to three foreign students a year. Dong Ching Chiu, a nineteen-year-old Chinese girl from Sarawak, came to be interviewed in pursuit of one of these scarce places.

Dong came from a family with medical leanings. Her grandfather was a headmaster who dabbled in Chinese medicine and her father had spent a term reading medicine at Taiwan University before switching to engineering. Now he was a civil engineer, married to a teacher of Chinese, and had dispatched his eldest daughter to boarding school in England at the age of fifteen. After excellent O level results and a grade A in art A level which she took at the same time, Dong Chiu chose to do A levels in Physics, Chemistry and Maths and when she visited St Mary's for her interview, she had just sat her exams. She was poised, elegantly dressed and strikingly attractive, with short, spiky, black hair and careful make-up.

Dong Chiu placed St Mary's top of her list of medical schools on the advice of her headmaster, who told her that the Dean had connections with Sarawak which might help her. She had thought of several alternatives to medicine – in particular, architecture, which would have given her an opportunity to exercise her considerable artistic talent – but in the end her love of science had won. She wanted to train in London because a British medical degree would be accepted anywhere in the world. She had already had an offer from Cardiff and interviews were in the pipeline at Nottingham and Newcastle. Dong often took a breathtakingly long time to answer questions, an unnerving trait which increased her aura of self-possession and hinted at a tantalising depth of character. She said she liked doing things with her hands and thought she might go into surgery. Eventually she wanted to return to Sarawak to practise. Quizzed about her weaknesses, she replied, 'I think perhaps I take things too seriously. I want to get everything perfect, and sometimes I get disappointed if I don't. If I couldn't help somebody I might get upset. But I wouldn't show it; I tend to hide things that are not right to show.'

The usual questions about hobbies and interests yielded not only such conventional accomplishments as singing and playing the piano rather well, but also a liking for Tai Chi, which she described as a 'gentle' Chinese martial art. St Mary's was close to art galleries, which she loved. Her parents had assured her they would support her throughout medical school.

Immediately after the interview, Dong Chiu giggled with relief, but was unsure what kind of impression she had made. 'They didn't look very pleased with me, I feel. I stumbled over my words and I was a bit monotonous in the way I spoke. I was so nervous that I couldn't think properly. The worst question was, why do you want to be a doctor? It is so difficult because you can't exactly put a list down: it brings in good pay, it's got good job prospects – that sounds very greedy. And the other bit of it, the interesting side, is so hard to explain.'

In fact, Dong Chiu had impressed the panel. One interviewer summed up their feelings when he remarked, 'I think she could be a high flier who could also adapt to the demands of clinical medicine. The whole question of being Chinese in Malaysia is a very tricky background. There's a depth there which I like.' Dong Chiu was offered a place conditional on getting a B and two Cs in her A levels and secured it with an A in physics and Bs in Maths and Chemistry. She rejected offers from Cardiff and Newcastle.

Professor Charles Easmon, who sat on Dong Chiu's panel, was a graduate of St Mary's himself and a veteran of the admissions procedure. He believed that the interview served a useful purpose, but acknowledged its limitations. 'With the competition for medical school places, we are looking to exclude those who, despite their intellectual ability, are totally incapable of establishing any sort of relationship with people, or haven't got the resilience to become a doctor.' Many of the independent school candidates exuded confidence, he said. 'Some of them sit down and almost start to interview us. This is much less common in those that have been to state schools, and we must take it into account, because it is easy to be misled by a veneer of sophistication and confidence.' None of the panel members were professional interviewers and Professor Easmon thought it inevitable that they would miss good people who might make very good doctors. 'It's a bit of a lottery, and whatever we do, we won't get it perfect, but in this school there is a constant attempt to refine and improve the procedures. What really makes the morning is a good, lively candidate who surprises you by going well above what you've seen on the application form. When that happens it's a revelation – and the interview system is working.'

The interview was vitally important for mature applicants, men and women who had studied or worked in another field for several years before opting for medicine. Some medical schools would not consider applications from mature students: few took students over the age of twenty-five and hardly anyone was accepted after the age of thirty. Mary's was more welcoming to latecomers to medicine and therefore attracted a large number of applications from older candidates. 'It is not a disadvantage to be a mature applicant to St Mary's provided that you have something to offer,' commented the Dean. The school was less interested in people who had applied for medicine in the first place, failed to make the grade, now had a mediocre degree in natural sciences and were trying for a second time without having done any public service or achieved excellence in any field. But mature students who might not even have been to university but had made a success of one career and now felt they had a contribution to make in medicine were very much the sort of people St Mary's was looking for. 'I don't mind whether their previous experience has been something allied to medicine, like nursing or physiotherapy, or something totally different, like running a British Rail station, working as a croupier, or playing in an orchestra. The important thing is that they have done what they were doing well and don't want to change because they've failed. They just have a mission to make a different contribution.'

Will Liddell was one of those who discovered his mission to do medicine relatively late. The son of a Hampshire farmer, he was educated at Eton and Oxford, where he read zoology, then did a masters degree in the technology of crop protection at Reading University. Idealism combined with a love of biological sciences propelled him into agricultural aid to the Third World. But while he was working with the Overseas Development Agency (ODA) on a crop protection project in Bolivia he began to have doubts about spending his whole life as an agricultural scientist.

The turning point came during a holiday in the Hebrides in September, 1984, when he heard that a friend had started medicine at the age of 30. 'I suddenly thought: I could do that. I had wanted to do medicine when I was at school, but was told that it would be difficult as I had not got an A level in physics [Will got an A in Geography, and Bs in biology and chemistry], and at the time I wasn't motivated enough to pursue it. I immediately telephoned Edinburgh University from a booth on the beach and asked if I could visit them on my way home from the Hebrides to talk about doing medicine. Medicine seemed to combine everything that I wanted: meeting people, applied science and a feeling of self-worth. I wanted to have a job which I wouldn't have to question.'

Will resigned from the ODA and found a job as an auxiliary nurse at the Radcliffe Hospital, near his home in Oxford. Then he set about discovering which schools were interested in taking mature students. Bristol was his first choice, followed by four London hospitals. His first interview was at St Mary's and Will was terrified: 'I had been to a fair few interviews in the past, but I had never been as nervous as I was then: I felt cold and shaky. I had never been at an interview where so much was at stake. I wanted to get into medicine so badly and at the time Mary's was the only interview I had been offered and I thought it might be my only chance. I was shown round by a mature student, a man of twenty-nine who had been a teacher and was really enjoying life at Mary's. I found that really reassuring and it strengthened my conviction that I was doing the right thing.'

A slightly built man who looked less than his twenty-six years, with a mobile, intelligent face, concerned brown eyes and a hint of Hampshire in his vowels, Will faced a formidable selection panel. Chairman Dr George Tait and Professors Richard Beard

and George Brent pounced on the letter he had pinned to his
application form, in which he explained his reasons for wanting
to change career. They pointed out an apparent contradiction
between his interest in biological sciences and his desire to care
for people and eventually become a GP. Will's rueful admission
that he had 'tacked that bit on the end' won sympathetic laughter.
Professor Beard was worried that he would find the medical school
course frustrating and might not cope with being with much
younger students. Will said he thought he could.

The crunch question came from Professor Brent. 'How do you
defend yourself from the suggestion that you might have the
elements of the eternal student in you?' Will swayed in his seat
like a boxer who had spotted an upper cut coming. 'This is
something that I'm very sensitive about and I find it difficult to
defend myself,' he replied, explaining that he saw medicine as a
vocation and was willing to sacrifice several years in order to train
as a doctor. By the end of the interview the panel appeared
genuinely interested in Will, asking his views on the current
famine in Ethiopia ('it's about ideology and weather, not agri-
culture') and the effects of inflation in Bolivia. His interview was
much longer than average – about twenty-two minutes – but he
appeared fairly comfortable. His gestures were confident and he
achieved an impressive combination of articulacy, candour and
humility.

The panel was split. Professor Brent was worried that Will had
not thought through his reasons adequately. Professor Beard came
to his defence: 'With all these mature students there is an element
of chance, but I would support him.' In the end they decided to
take a chance on Will and a few weeks later he was 'very, very
pleased indeed' to receive an offer from St Mary's, conditional
on him passing physics O level.

What did Will, veteran of many interviews, think of the St
Mary's admissions procedure? Was fifteen minutes long enough
to decide whether a candidate was worth the investment of thousands of pounds and capable of becoming a good doctor? 'The
interview system is not ideal,' Will said, in retrospect, 'but it's
much better than simply looking at A level results. After all, you
can tell a lot about someone in ten minutes and one of the things

you are trained to do at medical school is to size people up very quickly. For the doctors on the panel the fifteen minute interview is much longer than they have to assess a patient in an average out-patient clinic.'

Will Liddell was fortunate in that he faced no financial hardship. As a graduate he did not qualify for a grant. But just before he applied to St Mary's an elderly relative had died, leaving him a substantial legacy. There was enough to buy a flat close to St Mary's and to cover his living expenses as a student. 'Great-aunt Elsie made it all possible,' commented Will. 'I couldn't have asked my parents for any further support, and I would not have been able to think of entering medicine if it hadn't been for her.'

Unlike Will, most mature students have to make huge sacrifices, both financial and emotional. John Shephard, for example, had a wife, a mortgage and a promising career in the merchant navy when he was suddenly seized with a determination to become a doctor at the age of twenty-seven.

John came from a medical family. The son of a GP and a theatre sister, he grew up in a rambling house in the country which was also his father's surgery and where the dining room doubled as a waiting room. One of his cousins was a professor in Aberdeen, another specialised in tropical medicine, his godfather was a consultant anaesthetist and his uncle ran the medical services in one of the Gulf states. John went to King's School, Gloucester, where he took a handful of O levels, mostly in arts subjects. He describes his schoolboy self as 'a yob who kicked against the system' and when he left school at sixteen, his headmaster commented, 'We believe that he has intelligence, but we have been unable to unearth it.' John turned to the sea, entering the merchant navy as a navigating cadet. Three years later he joined the Royal Fleet Auxiliary, rising to the rank of Senior Second Officer, and serving with the United Nations Peacekeeping Force during the evacuation of Beirut in 1982.

In 1977, when he was twenty, he married Debbie, who had been his girlfriend for two years, and she often sailed with him on postings. During this period John studied for A levels in English and economics by correspondence with the quaintly named College of the Sea. He also took the week-long medical course that was compulsory for all officers of his rank, enabling them to act as ship's doctors, dealing with minor medical problems while the ship was at sea. Suddenly he was hooked. 'It was fascinating, and I wanted to know more. Most officers didn't like being ship's doctor, so I did it on three ships, over a period of about two years. By the end I was enjoying it more than my normal duties, which I found increasingly monotonous.' John was not involved in the Falklands War, but he lost four friends on the *Sir Galahad*, an experience which strengthened his growing conviction that medicine, rather than warfare, was his true métier.

The idea that he should change direction completely came from Debbie, who persuaded him that she could support them both while he studied for the necessary science A levels. She was also prepared to cope with long separations if he managed to find a place at medical school. So in 1984 John resigned from the Navy and began a one-year A level course at Plymouth College of Further Education, studying Physics, Chemistry and Biology. It was a terrible grind for a man who had done very little science, and none since the age of sixteen. Debbie meanwhile took a job as an estate agent in order to pay the mortgage on their rambling Victorian house on the outskirts of Plymouth. John topped up their income by navigating cross-Channel ferries whenever he had time during weekends and holidays.

He applied to medical schools during this A level year, placing Birmingham first and St Mary's second; Charing Cross, the London Hospital and Bristol were his other choices. St Mary's was the first school to interview him and he felt that the panel, chaired by the Dean, gave him an easy ride. 'I had an extremely good interview which lasted around ten minutes. I felt that they had already made up their minds to make me an offer and simply wanted to see what I looked like.' The man who sat facing the panel was tall and lean, with the short hair, blue eyes and clean-cut good looks of an Identikit naval officer. His authoritative manner and penetrating gaze suggested that he might not suffer fools gladly, and made him an unusual interviewee. He was keen to convince them of his dedication, especially since he would have less time to give back to the NHS once qualified, and made it clear that he knew what he was letting himself in for: he was not a man who shrank from hard work.

Two days after his interview John received an offer from St Mary's conditional on him getting three Cs in his A levels. He accepted, turning down offers from Birmingham and the London Hospital. The following August he was in the Mediterranean delivering a yacht when Debbie telephoned to say that he had not made the grades, obtaining only Ds in chemistry and biology. 'I was panic stricken, because I couldn't get in direct contact with St Mary's and I wanted them to hold the place open for me while I retook my A levels. In the end I wrote to them and they replied saying that they would take me despite my grades.' At 28 he was the oldest student admitted to Mary's in the 1985 intake.

John Shephard, the merchant seaman with no degree and indifferent A level grades, was able because of his naval background to prove that he possessed decision-making skills that are vital in medicine. Peter Richards, the Dean, stressed the importance of such qualities when he described what St Mary's looks for in its students. 'Humanity must be very high on the list, and intelligence, which isn't simply a matter of academic ability. It is the capacity to put knowledge into action. Medicine is about making decisions on incomplete evidence, changing them in the light of experience, and sometimes living with the consequences of your wrong decisions. And a substantial number of people who are very, very bright and very good academically are simply unable to cope with making decisions.' Most of the St Mary's intake consisted of school leavers, conventionally academic high achievers with wide interests. But every year Peter Richards helps a few less orthodox applicants to slip through the net. 'Each year I have one or two deliberate risks, who I have taken on hunch as people, even though academically they don't shine. Some do tremendously well and others are terrible disasters – but I keep my eye on them. I never reveal who they are.'

John Shephard is convinced that he was one of the Dean's wild cards. So too is Fey Probst, another mature student who went to enormous lengths to realise her long-cherished dream of winning a place at medical school. And for Fey the obstacles were considerable: she was the mother of four children and her marriage, to all intents and purposes, was over.

The ninth of ten children of a Greek engineer and his English wife, Fey grew up in Canada, Pakistan and Cornwall and decided at the age of eight that she wanted to be a doctor. She fell victim, however, to her academic precocity. She attended Millfield School, where she passed her A levels at sixteen – two years ahead of most contemporaries and far too young to apply to medical schools, which normally insist that students are at least eighteen on admission. Instead Fey sat Oxford entrance exams and won a place at Brasenose College to read biochemistry. But, like John Shephard, she was a rebel and just after her eighteenth birthday, to the fury of her parents, she married a computer programmer ten years her senior whom she had known since early childhood, and left Oxford.

During the next six years Fey had three children, two girls and a boy, and was a full-time mother. She loved looking after them, but never abandoned her hopes of a medical career. In 1983 when she finally started to apply for medical schools, she discovered that her A level grades were now too low. She was interviewed at the London Hospital, St Thomas's and Bristol, but received no offers. So she signed up for evening classes, first in physics, which she passed with a B while five months pregnant with Stephen, her fourth child, and later in chemistry, which she also passed with a B, when he was eight months old.

The following year, now aged twenty-six, she reapplied to medical school and was given an interview at St Mary's just before Christmas. The Dean chaired her interview panel. Fey was an extraordinary character: sharp and immensely confident with a pale, clever face, darting, watchful eyes, short fair hair and a degree of self-belief more commonly found in public school boys than housewives with small children.

'This time I had worked out the answers they wanted to hear,' recalled Fey. 'So when they said "Does your husband support you?" I said, "He gives me as much support as I need", even though we were living apart by then, because I knew I didn't need any support. They asked me why we had two addresses and

I implied it was because we were rather well off. I didn't lie, but I revealed only selective bits of the truth.'

When it came, the offer was unconditional and it said simply, 'Merry Christmas – a place is on offer.' Fey remembers, 'I was so elated – it was very hard to scrape me off the ceiling.'

A year after the interviews, the ten applicants returned to Mary's as medical students. In his welcoming lecture, the Dean told them, 'You are the survivors. Your presence here is a mixture of talent and luck. There were more than twenty-two applicants for each place you are now sitting in – and that is a jolly good reason for using your opportunity well.'

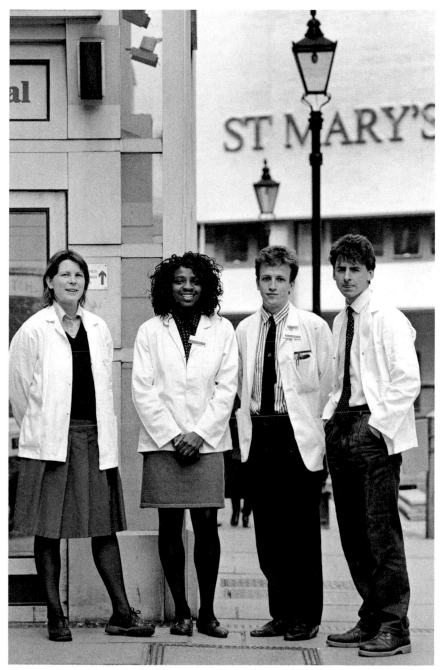

New clinical students: from left, Fey Probst, Ese Oshevire, David Copping and Will Liddell in their third year when they came into contact with patients for the first time.

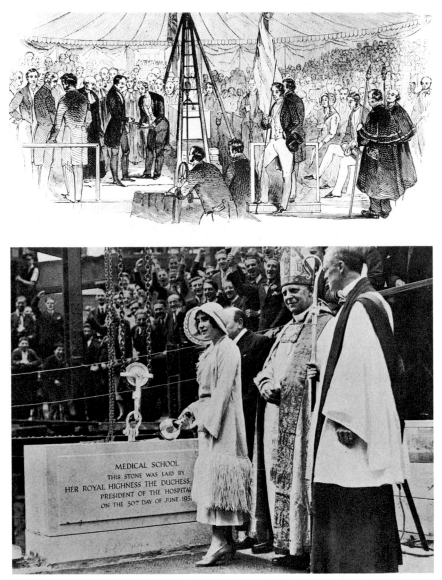

The royal connection: (top) in 1845 Prince Albert laid the foundation stone of St Mary's Hospital; (above) in 1931 the Duchess of York (now the Queen Mother) performed the same ceremony at the new medical school. Opposite he Queen's gynaecologist, Sir George Pinker, was a consultant at St Mary's and Princes William and Harry were both born in the private Lindo Wing. In 1982 waiting crowds caught their first glimpse of Prince William as the Prince and Princess of Wales left the hospital.

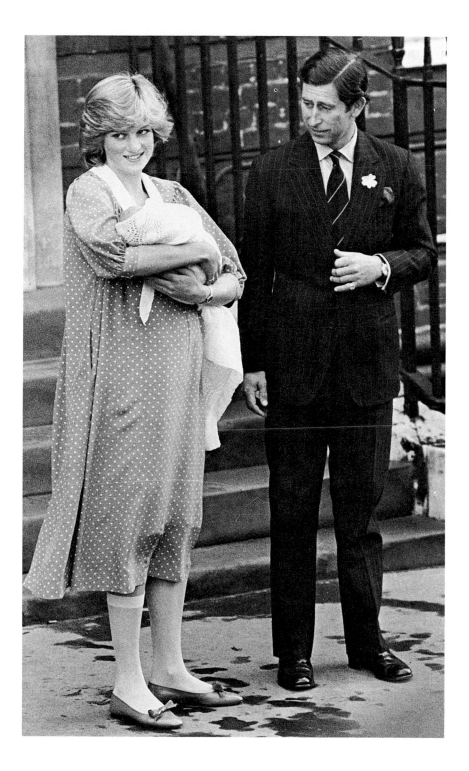

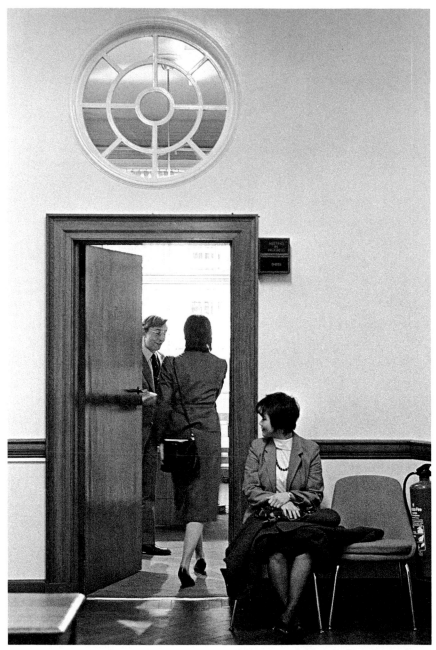

Waiting to face the panel: Dong Ching Chiu outside the medical school committee room before her admissions interview. St Mary's had twenty-two applicants for each of its places during the year she applied.

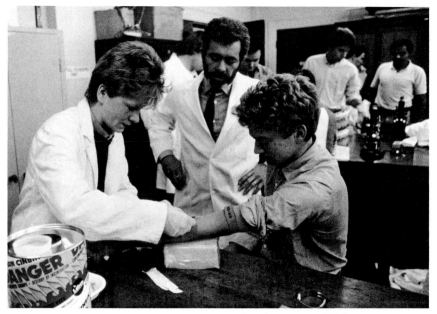

Students spend their first two years attending lectures and laboratory practicals. Above *Sarah Holdsworth learns to take blood from Nick Hollings during a physiology practical.* Below *Students get to grips with a skeleton during one of the anatomy sessions.*

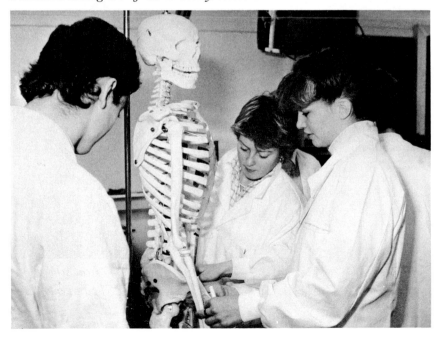

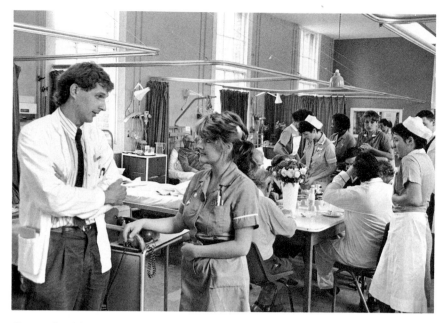

From the third year, students begin work as apprentice doctors, participating in the routine of wards (above, *John Shephard*) *and learning the rudiments of surgery in the operating theatre* (below).

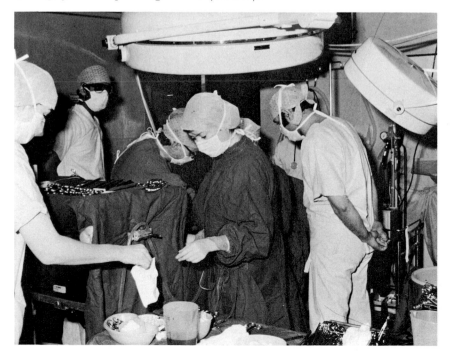

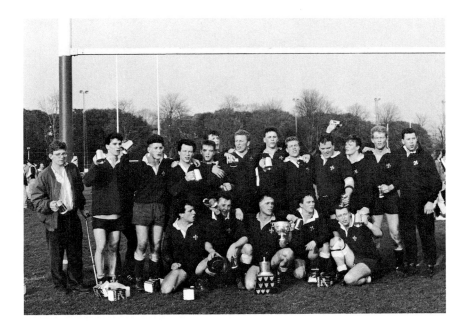

St Mary's students enjoy a wide range of extra-curricular activities. Rugby is still a dominant feature of life at the medical school and the 1st XV is a frequent winner of the Interhospitals Cup: (above) *the victorious team, 1991. Music and drama are equally strong: in 1989 Jane Morris and Sarah Holdsworth* (below, *second and third from left) directed and starred in the annual soiree – a two-hour medical cabaret.*

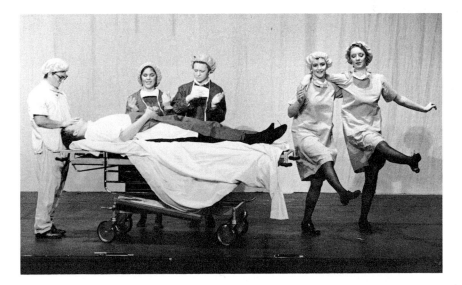

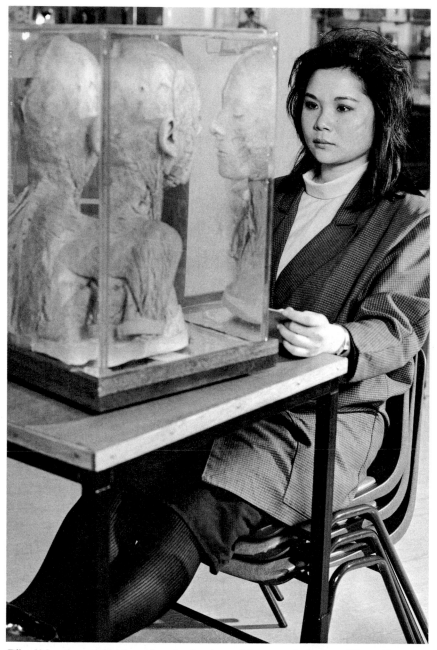

The life of a medical student is dominated by examinations. Here, Dong Ching Chiu revises before her first-year anatomy paper.

2

FIRST DAYS

On an unseasonably hot October afternoon in 1985, St Mary's Hospital Medical School greeted the 101 survivors of its selection process. The Dean had invited the new students and their parents to tea, and now they arrived in small family groups, each spearheaded by a diffident fresher. Dress was formal: suits and frocks; the atmosphere hovered somewhere between a school speech day and a garden party. Entering Norfolk Place, the parents gazed up at the hospital and medical school, their faces a blend of pride and nervousness.

The families were about to enter one of the youngest and smallest of London's great Victorian medical schools; an institution whose history was written in the stones above their heads. On one side of the street stood the old hospital, a large, elegant red-brick building whose foundation stone was laid by Prince Albert in 1845. The medical school was erected next to the hospital and admitted its first students in 1854. It grew steadily in size and prestige so that, by the 1920s, the original Victorian buildings were inadequate and money was raised to construct a new school. Queen Elizabeth the Queen Mother (who as Duchess of York and later Queen Elizabeth has had a sixty-year association with the school as its patron) laid the foundation stone in 1931 and two years later King George V opened the new medical school, an austere grey-brown building opposite the old hospital.

It housed laboratories, lecture theatres, a large library and a swimming pool.

Gathered in the medical school foyer with its polished wood, lofty ceiling and stone staircases were forty-six women and fifty-five men. Seven were mature students and four came from overseas. They came from all parts of England and Wales, but only one came from Scotland. Most were accompanied by both parents, but some came alone. Tea and sandwiches awaited them in the basement restaurant where parental reserve quickly gave way to the eager friendliness of strangers drawn together by common emotion and experience. Members of the medical school staff and older students circulated, dispensing tea and anecdotes.

The faces were overwhelmingly white, with a handful of Asians and just three black students, one of whom was Ese Oshevire. She was horrified when she realised that only a fraction of the students came from a background similar to hers. 'My foster-mother and foster-brother came to the tea party, and they noticed straight away how posh everyone was. I was surprised to discover how many people came from public schools and I could count on the fingers of two hands those people who came from social class 5. There were three black students in my year, and I thought there would be more than that.' Sarah Holdsworth was also surprised to find herself in a minority. 'Everyone seemed to have very posh accents and there were only five other people from the North.' For Dong Chiu, 20,000 km from home and unaccompanied by her parents, the first day was an ordeal. 'Before it all started I was very excited, but at the Dean's tea party I felt very lost. There was no one for me to lean on.' Most of the students, however, commented that the people they met at the tea party were similar to their school friends – they estimated that roughly eighty per cent of the year came from independent schools.

Peter Richards welcomed the parents. 'Many of you will have discovered already that, once children get to university, their parents don't matter any more – at least, not until money runs short. But the course here is tough, there are many stresses and strains, and I think your offspring will need your support.' He referred bleakly to problems faced by the universities and the health service: 'The financial future looks very grim indeed and there is rough water ahead – both for hospital and school – but we shall do everything to ensure that the education of our students and service to our patients does not suffer.'

After the tea party most students returned to Wilson House, an accommodation block ten minutes' walk from the medical school in Sussex Gardens. Bought by the school in 1949, it was originally twenty large Victorian terrace houses which were converted into bedsitting rooms for half the students. A new sports hall and recreation centre had just been added. The rooms were small and plain, but they were central, cheap and coveted: rents in London were beyond the pockets of many students. Posters, plants, cushions and rugs quickly transformed the smallest, darkest room into a satisfactory first home.

Wilson House was the scene of a party thrown by St Mary's Students' Union that evening. Last goodbyes had been said to families, and smart clothes discarded in favour of jeans and T-shirts. Older students handed out bread and cheese while the freshers elbowed their way into the crowd at the bar in pursuit of a drink. Introductions were shouted, A level grades compared, and anxieties pooled as the freshers began their search for the people who would be their friends for the next five or six years.

Sarah Holdsworth, Jane Morris and Ese Oshevire had met for the first time the day before, at a University of London hostel not far from Wilson House. That night they had seen prostitutes for the first time. 'I got back to my room very late on the first night and I was too excited to sleep, so I opened my window and sat looking out,' recalled Sarah. 'There were a lot of women walking down the road, all dressed up, and I wondered where they were going. Then I saw cars slowing down, and one by one they all got into the cars. I suddenly realised they must be prostitutes and I couldn't believe it; I was very shocked. I woke up the girl next door to tell her. She had never seen them before either and we both stayed up for hours watching them from my window.' Prostitutes used to ply their trade blatantly in Sussex Gardens, and female students were frequently accosted or pestered by kerb crawlers on their way to and from Wilson House. Today, in the wake of a clean-up operation by local police, there are fewer prostitutes on the streets of Paddington, but there is still a flourishing underground sex industry in the area, and the venereal disease clinic at St Mary's Hospital is one of the busiest in Europe.

The serious business of becoming a medical student began the following morning when everyone assembled in the physiology theatre, an old-fashioned steep-sided lecture theatre, for the Dean's introductory talk. It was a sombre affair, hinting at tough times ahead, and stiff penalties for those who fell from grace. 'St Mary's is not a rest home for tired A level performers,' he warned, scanning his audience through spectacles. 'We have great sympathy with difficulty and practically none with idleness. The saddest task I have each year is that of saying goodbye to students who have failed their first- or second-year exams.'

The use of drugs was absolutely prohibited and would result in instant expulsion with no appeal. If possible, they should refrain from smoking, for the sake of their own health and in order to set an example to their patients. Alcohol was fine in moderation, but they should beware: 'Alcoholism is common in the medical profession and, for many, the habit started as a student.'

The rest of the day was filled with speeches, explanations and introductions. Countless copies of the same passport size photograph had to be handed over to different people. Students had to register with the school, get hold of grant cheques, obtain library membership, join the St Mary's students' union and collect their University of London Union cards. And after lunch there was another lecture – with a difference.

The Norfolk Lecture was one of St Mary's traditions. It was a spoof lecture, which had been given every year for as long as anyone could remember for the benefit of newcomers, although, as usual, the gangways were packed with older students too. In 1985 the speaker was Dr David Thomas, consultant neurologist at St Mary's and a popular and diverting lecturer, resplendent in waistcoat, scarlet carnation and silk handkerchief. Beside him on a trolley sat a pyjama-clad 'patient', with a nurse as chaperone.

The humour was typical medical revue fare: rude and crude. A succession of first years were summoned from the audience to assist in the examination of the young male patient. One had to hold up a number plate to test the patient's sight; it said EEG 1 (a reference to the number plate of Dr Thomas's Rolls Royce) but the patient read PENI 5 – to roars of laughter. Another tested the patient's reflexes by applying a vibrator to his bare foot. The patient was copiously 'sick' (a convincing cocktail of water and chopped vegetables) over a girl who examined his throat too energetically, prompting Dr Thomas to stress the importance of white coats. David Copping was asked to find out whether diabetes was present by tasting a specimen of urine for its sugariness.

Jane Morris was another victim: she was invited to examine the patient, who removed his shirt to reveal a lacy black bra and suspender belt. 'Do you notice anything wrong with this patient?' demanded Dr Thomas. Jane shook her head. 'No? Well for Paddington that is quite normal,' he conceded and asked Jane to test the man's abdominal reflex with a sharp object. She used her fingernails and what began as an examination ended as a caress, with the patient beaming with pleasure.

The audience rocked with laughter throughout the lecture. Jokes which focus on the uncomfortable similarity between feeling someone's abdomen and stroking it for pleasure are perhaps especially potent for a group of people who spend their professional lives walking that tightrope every time they see a patient. For the older students in the audience, testing urine, genital examinations, questions about patients' sex lives, were all familiar territory. They laughed the loudest. The novices joined in, some with bewilderment, others with embarrassment. Their initiation was under way.

Hard on the heels of the spoof lecture came another, more serious, address. Dr Oscar Craig, consultant radiologist and elder statesman of St Mary's, led the newcomers through the five-year course, describing what was involved in each part. Here was a consultant straight out of *Doctor in the House*. A short, stocky showman in his late fifties, with comedian's eyes and slicked back brown hair, he kept up an extraordinary soliloquy for almost an hour and held his audience spellbound. He paced the stage, imitating the posture of medical students, shaking his fists, laughing, staring and pointing at them. His Irish brogue ran the entire histrionic gamut, from confidential whisper to falsetto shriek. It was a bravura performance.

He began by describing the different hospitals which they would visit during their studies. The course was centred on St Mary's, the great teaching hospital next to the medical school, but would also take them to St Charles' in the heart of Notting Hill, the Samaritan Hospital for Women in the Marylebone Road, the Central Middlesex in Park Royal and many other hospitals outside London.

'Not only are you lucky to be medical students, you are doubly or trebly lucky to be students at St Mary's. You have reason for the most fantastic pride.' Warming to his theme, Dr Craig told them about the great names of St Mary's. Augustus Waller, the physiologist who discovered the ECG and transformed the approach to heart disease. Almroth Wright, one of the founders of immunology. Alexander Fleming, one of Wright's pupils, who had discovered penicillin in the very building in which they now sat. Sir Bernard Spilsbury, England's greatest forensic scientist. The list grew longer and the claims larger. 'There have been more Fellows of the Royal Society at St Mary's Hospital than at any other hospital or medical school in these islands. Not only have we had all these academic distinctions, we've also had four captains of England at rugby, and one captain of Wales. We can do it all here. Be proud. Wear the tie with pride, wear the scarf with pride, wear the fleur de lys with pride.' A gold fleur de lys on a navy blue background is the symbol of St Mary's Hospital Medical School.

He went on to draw on the blackboard a 'graph of enthusiasm' which would reflect their changing attitudes to the course. Today, for example, there was a surge of pride and excitement as they stood on the threshold of their careers. 'This is one of the greatest days of your life. Are you aware of it? You are perched here, waiting for your whole life to be changed in a way nothing else can,' he told his audience.

'During the first year, it's great. You're in London, you're on your own. You've got pals – for the boys there are girls, for the girls there are boys. It all clicks.' But, he warned, initial excitement and euphoria would be followed by a chequered emotional career in which depression and self-doubt alternated with exhilaration.

'Does it take great brains to become a good doctor? I don't

think it does, you know. Does it take hard work? By George, it does! The work you have got to do is phenomenal. You've got to work harder and harder and harder.' They would have no time to march round Hyde Park carrying banners, but should, nevertheless, make time for the rich social, artistic and sporting life of the school. It was all a matter of getting the balance right.

Having dealt with the inner medical student, Dr Craig turned his attention to surface details. 'Patients – and patients are what this game is all about – like you to look like a doctor. And, from yesterday, you are all members of the medical profession. Immediately you start seeing patients, I for one will insist that the boys wear a tie. I don't want you on the ward in open-necked shirts. Now you might say to me, do you think that the way you're dressed makes you a better doctor? Let me assure you, it does, because your rapport with the patient is that much better.'

'You'll never have this lecture again,' he concluded. 'But please remember every word of it. The future of patients is in your hands. You've got a duty. You've got a price to pay for where you are and you've got to enjoy it. And I wish you the very best of luck.'

The students clearly enjoyed the lecture and appeared excited as they left the lecture theatre. Ese Oshevire summed up the feelings of many. 'He kept saying: you are the cream, and at times you believed it. He made us feel inspired to go on and do great things.' Sarah Holdsworth agreed. 'I felt full of pride. We all wanted to be doctors so much that time and he was brilliant. For me it was the high point of Freshers' Week.'

It was also, perhaps, the most significant event of the first few days. Dr Craig flattered the new entrants by hailing them as fellow professionals, and offering them an insider's view of the stresses, sacrifices and rewards of a medical career. More importantly, he stood before them, a high priest of the medical school, preaching its institutional values and celebrating its history and esprit de corps. He was making 'Mary's Men' – and women – of them.

Medical education has always been steeped in tradition and the contemporary curriculum is still based on a Victorian model. Tradition is nowhere more important than in the nine London undergraduate medical schools. They have very different characters, spawn fiercely loyal alumni, and compete for academic and athletic glory. Although St Mary's is a relatively young school (it was founded 731 years after Bart's), the concerns of its founding fathers powerfully influence the habits and values of today's teachers and students.

The spirit and character of St Mary's were largely the creation of the school's most illustrious Dean, Charles Wilson (later Lord Moran), physician and confidant to Winston Churchill. Soon after his arrival in 1920, Wilson decided to abolish the competitive entrance examination in favour of personal interviews with applicants recommended by the heads of university colleges and leading public schools. Sir Zachary Cope, who was professor of surgery during Wilson's time as Dean, summarised this new approach in his official history of St Mary's. 'He found that it was possible to select men of a very high standard of character and attainments. In this way there came to the school a considerable influx of students of high intelligence, outstanding character and considerable skill at games.'

Wilson loved sport – he once said, 'a good Dean is a man who will referee a Third XV game on a wet November Saturday afternoon' – and he forged St Mary's reputation, which persists to this day, as a centre of excellence for rugby. Several of the founding staff of St Mary's had been pupils of Dr Arnold at Rugby School and there had always been a strong interest in the sport, but from the 1930s onwards rugby became central to the school's culture. St Mary's has been the most frequent winner of the Interhospitals Rugby Cup during the post-war period and has produced scores of international players, among them Tommy Kemp and J.P.R. Williams. It has also been notably strong in athletics: Roger Bannister, hero of the sub-four minute mile, was a student and teacher at the medical school. Rugby is still the single most important sporting and social force at St Mary's. As a group medical students are taller than average, but in Paddington many of the men are huge. The school fields three teams and the annual cup final match, which almost invariably features the St Mary's first fifteen, empties the hospital and medical school for an afternoon every March. Students and consultants rub shoulders as they cheer their team to victory.

Wilson's determination to seek clever, characterful athletic men necessarily put female applicants at a disadvantage, but that too was in line with tradition: St Mary's had long been a bastion of anti-feminism. One of its most famous sons, Sir Almroth Wright, a bacteriologist and pioneer of vaccination, found fame among a wider public in 1913 with his pamphlet *The Unexpurgated Case against Women's Suffrage.*

During the First World War, many women entered medicine and in 1916 St Mary's grudgingly agreed to admit female students in order to provide clinical training for graduates of the London School of Medicine for Women in Hampstead. A women's common room was constructed and the wards and classrooms rapidly became co-educational. But one senses that the women were never made to feel at home among the rugger players of Paddington and in 1924 St Mary's decided to take no more of them. Zachary Cope reported that the numbers of female applicants had declined and that 'men, for the most part, preferred to go to a school where women were not taken'. The decision was reversed, however, in 1929, after the University of London said that it favoured co-education. The school wrote unenthusiastically to the university: 'St Mary's will be prepared to admit women students, provided that all metropolitan medical schools do the same.'

In 1947, London University insisted that all medical schools should ensure that at least fifteen per cent of their undergraduates were female. Until 1970, St Mary's operated an unofficial quota, limiting its intake of female students to twenty per cent of the total. Since then, the proportion has risen steadily and for the past eight years men and women have been admitted in roughly equal numbers. The teaching staff, however, remains overwhelmingly male and, despite the large numbers of female students, the place still has the atmosphere of a male institution.

When our students entered the school it was still an autonomous body, but five years earlier the University of London Senate had recommended that it should either close or merge with two other schools. St Mary's fought off that attempt on its life but in 1988 it merged, of its own accord, with the 5000-strong Imperial College, a national centre of scientific teaching and research situated on the opposite side of Hyde Park. The school's official title now became Imperial College of Science, Technology and Medicine, St Mary's Hospital Medical School. The merger safe-guarded the school's future while allowing it for the most part to retain its identity.

St Mary's is a small and extremely self-contained institution which seems still conscious of being a younger sibling among the London medical schools, anxious to prove that it can fend for itself, and can take on far larger institutions and win. There is a trace of siege mentality which produces terrific esprit de corps and forges friendships that last lifetimes, but can also induce feelings of claustrophobia.

During his time as dean, Peter Richards has sought to make the student body wider and more diverse and is credited with having widened St Mary's somewhat limited public image as a rugby players' paradise. He encouraged music and drama and severed the thread of nepotism which bound generations of Mary's men and led fathers to assume that their sons, irrespective of their intellectual calibre, would follow them as of right into the medical school. He could fairly claim to have enriched the culture. 'We simply try to take the best on their merits in open competition.'

On their third day at St Mary's, students underwent another initiation rite: their first visit to the anatomy dissection room, a prospect they regarded with a mixture of fascination and dread. Anatomy, the study of skeletons and cadavers, would take up a large part of the first two years of the course.

The first task for the class was to collect and sign for their half-skeletons, each housed in a brown cardboard box the length of an adult's thigh bone. The boxes were stacked against the rear wall from floor to ceiling, like the store room of a shoe shop. A human skeleton stood to attention next to the shelves. The students filed into the long room, stealing nervous glances at fifteen hospital trolleys covered with white plastic which lined the side walls. The irregular lumps underneath the plastic were the corpses which they would work on for the next eight months as they learned the art of dissection.

Involuntary sighs and whispered cries of 'Oh no' filled the room as they headed towards Vic Barber, the white-coated anatomy assistant who had worked in the department for seventeen years and introduced hundreds of students to the subject. 'They are a bit apprehensive at first when they go into the dissecting room,' he explained, 'but curiosity killed the cat, and they lift up a sheet and have a quick peep. It's not so bad because there are lots of them.' Vic issued each student with a set of dissecting instruments (a canvas pouch containing forceps, scalpels and scissors) and a skeleton number. Then they headed for the shoeboxes and pulled out their personal skeleton.

The year was divided into groups and Vic Barber took each group through a skeleton check. Seated on the floor, they opened their boxes and counted heads, hands, feet and all the bones in between. Every box contained a whole skull, plus half the normal complement of bones (from the right or left side of the skeleton). Each half-skeleton had belonged to a man aged between twenty-seven and thirty, and there were inevitably individual differences. 'He didn't clean his teeth very well,' commented one student, grimacing at her skull's broken and decayed jaw. Sarah Holdsworth's skeleton was so large that she mistook a hand for a foot. There was much hilarity, and the high-ceilinged room rang to Vic Barber's exhortations. 'Everybody find a clavicle. Have you all got one now? Miss Smith, you look a bit lost – have a good rake round in the box. That's it, well done! It's shaped a bit like a boomerang. Next, we have the humerus, or funny bone. ...'

Once the skeletons had been checked and returned to their boxes, the students moved to the trolleys for what, for most, was their first encounter with a corpse. They tended to approach in little groups and then the boldest would lift the drape and expose the stark, bleached body for a few seconds. Faces registered either shock or amusement, sometimes both. 'Look at his eyes, they're really strange.' 'It's really funny, it doesn't look like a body at all, it's all messy.' Second-year students were on hand to offer a closer look and explain what was involved in dissection. 'It's not as fiddly as with a rat,' commented one senior student brightly as she folded back the covers and described how they would begin by cutting the skin on the chest and pulling it back to expose the underlying muscles. The rest of the term would be spent slowly dissecting the chest, arm and hand.

In an introductory talk to the students later in the week, Prof. Aidan Breathnach recalled the dark days of murder and grave robbing which preceded the 1832 Anatomy Act. 'We've come a long way since the days of Burke and Hare. You can no longer sell your body for dissection, and neither, if you are murdered, will anatomists buy your body. Every cadaver here is bequeathed, before death, by that individual and without that generosity the anatomy teaching which you would get would be very poor. So do realise, as you are doing your dissection, that you are benefiting from the goodwill and generosity of someone who has died and bequeathed their body to you.'

Dong Chiu found her first sight of cadavers both frightening and fascinating. 'I felt a sense of awe. I remember vividly the little hairs on the skin which brought the bodies to life, otherwise they were pallid and dead. I thought it was very good of those people to donate their bodies and I decided to leave mine to medicine.'

The whole afternoon was a most effective bonding exercise for the year. All went in nervous, uncertain what they would see and how they would react, and they laughed and learned together. The standard first aid lecture had the same effect. Students all had a turn at mouth-to-mouth resuscitation and cardiac massage. The lecturer explained that they were taught the basics of resuscitation so that they would be able to help if an emergency arose. The techniques were hard to master and everyone had to have a go while the others watched.

The social round continued with a Meet the Tutors cheese and wine party in the medical school canteen. The tutors were drawn from the teaching staff and five or six students were assigned to each one. The system was designed to provide pastoral care and some students found the arrangement extremely useful, visiting their tutors regularly for advice and help. Others were disappointed. 'I met mine once,' said David Copping, 'and that was it. He had obviously been forced to be a tutor and hated it. The system can work well: some tutors take their students to dinner, drinks and the theatre and hold regular meetings which can be very interesting. The trouble is, it's very variable.'

Most of the tutors were men and they were identifiable by their ties. Little groups of students gathered round the ties. One tutor asked his group what they were most looking forward to. Dissection on Monday, was the unanimous answer. 'We want to see who makes the first cut.' 'And who passes out first.' The round of receptions and parties was already beginning to take its toll. 'This first week is so … baffling,' as one student put it.

In an attempt to reduce the levels of bewilderment induced by the variety and pace of life at St Mary's, the students' union organises a Link-Up meeting during the first week, at which each fresher is paired with two 'parents' – older students from the second and fourth years. The idea is that the second year shows the novice around the medical school, helps with the settling-in process and explains the course work in the first two years, while the fourth year organises a tour of the hospital and introduces the student to wards and patients for the first time. Several students suggested that the most important part of the relationship was the loaning of lecture notes to freshers – a practice which is discouraged by the authorities, but much appreciated by the recipients since it means they can miss the occasional lecture with impunity. Some students made friends with their 'parents' and gained a great deal, others found themselves abandoned after a perfunctory first meeting.

Perhaps in recognition of risks attendant upon the hectic social life offered to newcomers, many of whom had been used to a more restricted life either in the bosom of their families or at boarding school, one of the earliest lectures was on the subject of contraception. Much giggling and whispering preceded the arrival of the speaker, Mr David Paintin, a gynaecologist clad in a white coat, who introduced himself as the person who would co-ordinate teaching on human sexuality during their five years at medical school. 'I am also here because there are people in the medical school who have a neurotic worry that, unless I talk to you on your first morning, you will all be pregnant by Christmas,' he added. Much laughter.

He warned that, now they were medical students, friends would regard them as experts on the subject of contraception and would sidle up to ask their advice about different methods. 'Doctors need to be sexually mature themselves if they are to going to help patients with these problems. And sex looms surprisingly large in every doctor's practice.' Quite so, but at the moment they were medical rookies, and sexually they were probably years behind their peers. 'In terms of sexual behaviour, you're likely to be a moderately retarded group. You've been working hard for your A levels over the past two or three years, and you've not been so much out in the world as other people in your age group. Seventy per cent of men, and fifty per cent of women have had heterosexual experience by the age of eighteen, but the figures are probably much lower in the group here today.' The unspoken implication was that, with A levels finally over, the students might have a lot of catching up to do, especially in their first delicious weeks of liberty ...

David Paintin managed to communicate serious messages about responsible sexual behaviour by addressing his audience as fellow-professionals. Homosexuality was a 'normal variant' of sexual behaviour, he said. Sexual morality was a private matter and the medical school would not dream of making rules about it. They should behave according to the moral code that had evolved out of their upbringing and experience. It was often difficult for individuals to resist peer group pressure to be sexually active, but such pressure should be resisted: 'people should only do these things if it is proper and right for them at the time'. Poorly controlled sexual behaviour could be harmful and might leave a 'permanent bruise' in the form of psychological damage, venereal disease or an unplanned pregnancy. Good quality relationships generally avoided these hazards, but casual sex resulted in the spread of disease and the risk of abortion. Proper communication between couples was the key to a successful relationship. 'I'm deliberately not talking about contraception in detail. It is knowing you need it that's important!'

At the end of his lecture, Mr Paintin asked for questions. There was a long, embarrassed silence, broken by an inquiry about the new 'morning-after' pill. Then everyone shuffled out of the lecture theatre. Looking back on the lecture several years later, most students felt that it had been both useful and necessary. 'People went quite wild during the first few weeks,' remembered one girl. 'There was a party every night for the first fortnight and most of us just weren't used to it. Quite a lot of pairing off went on.'

The medical school authorities knew that, while experimenting with their new-found freedom, students might overlook the fact that they had embarked upon a highly demanding academic course. In his first lecture Professor Breathnach reminded them of their responsibilities. 'You are the élite, a highly selected group to which the nation has seen fit to hand its healthcare.' But he warned that now they were at medical school, their methods of learning would have to change radically. The spoon-feeding of knowledge to which they had grown accustomed in their sixth forms was now at an end. 'At school you were taught with the object of getting here as medical students, against stiff competition. Now the onus is much more on you: you are now adults, and so it is extremely difficult for us to force you to learn.'

The students were already aware that a great deal of work lay ahead. Sarah Holdsworth voiced the feelings of many when she said, 'I think it will be tough, but I like a challenge and I shall have to last the course – my parents will never let me live it down if I don't.' Mark George was concerned about the end of year exams. 'I'm worried about passing my first year. It is very, very competitive. There might be times when I'm pretty narked off with medicine, but I think I'll stick it.' Dong Chiu was also worried about the exams, because she had not taken biology A level and feared that she might get left behind in some subjects. Will Liddell, one of the mature students, felt more confident. 'I think the work is going to be a pretty severe load, but having done a degree already I think I have the advantage of being able to organise myself well from the beginning.'

Fey Probst was an object of amazement to the other first years. They could not believe that anyone could undertake the volume of work which faced them all and raise a family. Fey admitted that it was tough, but she was typically philosophical. 'It's very difficult to look after four children whether you're starting on a medical course or not. I have a fantastic nanny during the day, but when I get home I have to cope with the children, the washing up, the dinner and any academic work I have to do as well. I think there will be a lot of work. I'm hoping to fit it all into two evenings a week and a bit at weekends, leaving me three evenings a week and most weekends with the children.'

Fey received a full grant to cover her living expenses, but found clothing and feeding her children was a considerable drain on her resources. She had already started to attend any lunchtime meetings which provided food, in order to secure a free lunch for herself and to whisk away any sandwiches left over at the end that might do for supper. When staff at the medical school learned of her circumstances, several lecturers and registrars brought in bags of outgrown children's clothes and she reckoned that half the family's wardrobe came from this source over the next few years.

Most of the students received grants from their local authorities which paid their tuition fees, and some were eligible for maintenance grants which covered their living expenses. The size of the grants varied according to parental income. For students in London a full grant was £2845 a year during the pre-clinical course and £4033 during the clinical course (1991 values). In 1990 a gradual phasing out of grants began, in the face of great hostility from medical schools and their students; the grant was frozen, but could be topped up by low-interest loans. In 1991 students whose parents earned more than £32 000 received no maintenance grant at all: their parents were expected to make up the full value of the grant. Roughly half the students at St Mary's fell into this category.

As soon as they arrived at medical school, many students began to look for jobs which would help supplement their grant. Ese Oshevire found work as a waitress in a nearby hotel. She did a couple of eight-hour sessions per week; it was hard work, but she needed the money. John Shephard continued to pilot cross-channel ferries at weekends and during holidays in order to help pay the bills for his house in Plymouth. Sarah Holdsworth sold double glazing over the phone – and was so good at it that the company offered her a full-time job as a telephone sales supervisor. Many students took part in drug trials where they acted as guinea pigs for new products in return for cash. London, they discovered, was expensive and no one seemed to be able to survive on the basic grant.

Temptations to play were everywhere. A blackboard in the foyer urged everyone to audition for the chorus in a forthcoming production of *Half a Sixpence*. Alongside it was a stand where officers of the students' union were selling tickets for a 'toga party'. The Four-Legged Stagger Round Paddington was advertised on notice boards throughout the medical school and drew a large and exotic entry of male and female students from all years, including the freshers. The stagger was the kind of organised pub-crawl that constitutes a rite of passage in many British undergraduate communities, involving a great deal of beer, vomit and raucousness.

Teams crowded into the medical school bar, clad in a variety of bizarre costumes to the cheers of the other students. One trio wore surgical gowns, heavily bandaged heads and faces, and dark glasses. Another peered out at the opposition through stocking masks and black binliners. Several of the men were dressed as transvestites. The names of the runners were chalked up on a blackboard (Wee Willie Winkle and Pulling Power were typical entries) and the organiser leapt on to a table to explain the rules. 'Pint here, pint in the Fleming, pint in the Recreation Centre, then the Standard, the Exchange, and back here. Any order you like, but you've got to check in with the people with check boards. Males must drink six pints of ale and girls three pints.' He then gave a graphic demonstration of how to vomit into a bucket.

One team gave a brief summary of the point of the exercise before setting off. 'In theory, you go to the pubs, down six pints as quickly as possible and attempt to break the record, which is around twelve minutes. In practice, after the second pint, you may need to go for the odd fingers down the throat, bring up what you can and then keep going on a slightly empty stomach. It pays not to have too much in your stomach.' With that they set off into the night, shouts of 'Right, left, right, left!', interspersed with rugger chants, echoing through the dark, wet streets of Paddington.

There was a winning team, but playing the game was definitely more important than breaking the record, and a good time seemed to be had by all. One competitor summed it up. 'It was very hard. We were sick as parrots. We've only got one pint left – the other five pints are decorating Paddington. We shall definitely try again next year.'

In fact, the Four-Legged Stagger never took place again: the following year the Dean banned it. 'I thought the event was quite incompatible with a serious institution – especially one concerned with health,' he commented.

The Freshers' Fayre was a more restrained affair. St Mary's boasted more than forty clubs and societies, each of which had set up a stall in the Sports Hall dedicated to the pursuit of new members. There was everything from a wine society to a madrigal group. Nick Hollings and David Copping joined the fencing club. Ese signed up for almost everything, but in the end devoted most time to the Catholic Society (she became president the following year) and the Athletics Club. Jane and Sarah joined the ski club, Will Liddell joined the Boat Club and the Mountaineering Club and Mark George signed up to play hockey.

By the end of Freshers' Week most of the new students were nursing substantial hangovers and suffering from entertainment exhaustion but they had developed a sense of belonging and a year-identity. Many had already acquired partners. Jane Morris had auditioned for, and secured, one of the three female parts in the Christmas play and had started going out with one of her fellow actors – a student in the year above – who was to be her boyfriend for the next four years. Ese, who had known no one at first, made friends quickly during the endless parties and events, but was glad when it all finished. 'It got a bit stupid towards the end, we ran out of things to say to one another.' She too had met her future boyfriend, Simon Stacey, another first year. They had been brought together by their commitment to Christianity and a mutual love of reggae music.

For Dong Chiu the initiation rites were a trial. 'I was fairly miserable for the first few weeks and only went to one evening event. I don't like large gatherings of people I don't know and didn't go on any of the pub crawls, so I didn't make many friends. I tend to be the introvert type, so it was quite hard to see all these strangers and go up to them and chat. There's a lot of socialising in the first few days and I feel there is a real pressure to join lots of events. I didn't fit in at all.' Dong joined several organisations such as Amnesty International, Third World First and the Photographic Society, but admitted that none of them involved much socialising. She also did a great deal of costume and make-up for many plays and musicals and designed posters for a variety of clubs and several covers of the *St Mary's Gazette* – the journal of the medical school which was published every term.

David Copping felt that St Mary's had exceeded his expectations. 'I'm in a very friendly year and they seem a nice bunch, though very public school. I made friends very quickly, particularly with people whose names began with C, because we are always grouped together alphabetically for classes. Every year there is a rugby weekend, before term begins, for all the first year men who are interested in playing rugby. They have trials for the team, and generally get to know one another. Many of the men in my year had been to it, and for my first term I felt a bit out of things because I wasn't a "rugger bugger", as they are known. They are very cliquey and it can be a bit intimidating if you are not involved, but when you meet them on their own, they are very approachable people.' David joined the Christian Union in Freshers' Week and soon became involved in many of its activities.

For mature students like Will Liddell the frenetic socialising of Freshers' Week was less of a novelty, but he was pleased to have chosen St Mary's. 'Any medical school would have been difficult to adjust to, because I'm having to go back a stage in my career, but Mary's does have a number of other graduate students and it makes things easier when you've got someone to talk to who is facing similar readjustment problems.'

Most of the school leaver entrants were vague about their long-term future in medicine. All were sure that they would practise as doctors, but none knew where they would end up. Some of the mature students, in contrast, had already begun to make plans. Fey confidently predicted, 'In ten years' time I'll probably be a consultant, or working my way up to being one, and probably in surgery, which I've always had most interest in, ever since I was little. I shan't ever regret my decision to enter medicine and I'm sure I shall last the course. I've already dropped out of university once and I don't intend to do it again.'

John Shephard thought he would head in the opposite direction. 'I would like to go into general practice. At my age I'm too old to be a specialist and I think contact with people is the important thing. And I'd like to work in the kind of areas where there are square miles per doctor, rather than doctors per square mile.' He too was sure that he would manage to qualify: 'I certainly intend to last the course. I've given up too much not to get through now.'

3

LEARNING THE BASICS

Once the excitement and excess of Freshers' Week had come to an end, the new students had to settle down to some real work. The medical course at St Mary's followed a traditional British pattern which was was laid down at the beginning of the last century, when an act of Parliament established basic requirements for the training of doctors. It stipulated that practitioners should have completed a five-year apprenticeship, attended lectures on anatomy, physiology, theory and practice of medicine, pharmacology and chemistry, passed an oral examination and worked for six months in a hospital.

In 1985 our students, like their Victorian predecessors, were preparing for five years of study. Their course was divided into two parts: the first two years, known as the pre-clinical course, consisted of lectures and practicals in basic medical sciences, which were taught at the medical school. The next three years were devoted to clinical medicine, literally the study of illness and disease in patients, which took them into the hospital.

The pre-clinical phase was designed to teach students the minimum they needed to know before being let loose on patients. The two years were dominated by examinations which took place each June. At the end of the first year students were examined in seven subjects. If they failed, they had to resit the exams in the following September. Those who failed again had to leave St Mary's. The second-year exams covered fourteen subjects. Again, students were allowed only two attempts at the examination and any who failed the September resits had to give up medicine. The importance of this timetable scarcely needed to be explained to the students; the exams created their own pressure, an ever-present, never-forgotten, much talked about enemy. Some students worked hard throughout their pre-clinical years; others saved their sweat until the term before the exams. But the knowledge that failure could mean the end of their medical career was with them all the time. It surfaced in a hectic social life culminating in events like Rag Week, strategically positioned halfway through the academic year.

Our students discovered that their days – unlike those of most undergraduates – were timetabled and that they were expected to work from nine to five every day, with a half hour break in the morning and an hour off for lunch, attending lectures, tutorials and practical sessions in the laboratory. The volume of work was large, and the teaching was significantly different from anything they had experienced before. More than half their time during the first two years was spent in lectures. Most took place within the medical school, in old-fashioned tiered lecture theatres dating from the 1930s. The whole year attended lectures together, peering down at blackboard and lecturer and scribbling frantically for an hour at a time. The remaining hours were split between practicals (around one and a half days a week) and tutorials.

Anatomy dominated the first year, initially because students were scared and excited at the prospect, later because so much of their time was taken up trying to learn the subject. During the first year the course revolved around the gradual dissection of a whole body. In his introductory lecture the professor of anatomy, Aidan Breathnach, told the students what was required of them. 'Once you get used to it, dissection is not difficult, we are not expecting you to produce marvellous dissections, the main thing is to reveal the parts you are supposed to reveal and to understand what you see.'

He urged them to make good use of the skeletons they had been given. 'I must impress upon you the value of the bones – which provide you with landmarks which allow you to relate the soft parts of the body to each other and to the bones. Before you come to dissect each part, try to read up on the bones the night before. In the oral exam in June, you will be questioned on the skeleton. During the war when we were students, we were cold because we didn't have any fuel and we took to studying in bed, and one could even bring one's bones to bed. We would have a humerus [upper arm bone] underneath the bedclothes, having learned it, and we could, by touch, test out our knowledge – not a bad way to learn your anatomy.

'This term you are doing the upper limb, the thorax, and beginning on the head and neck. Next term the head and neck and the abdomen and in the final term, the lower limb. So try and settle into a routine of regular study throughout the week.'

The weekly dissection classes were attended by the whole year. Gathering all hundred students together possibly made it easier for them to overcome their natural inhibitions about cutting into dead human flesh. With the whole group engaged in the activity, it was, curiously enough, more comfortable for individuals to conform and get on with it than to run away in revulsion.

There were fifteen cadavers for the year and students were divided into groups of seven or eight. Groups were responsible for keeping their cadavers in good condition and members took turns at dissection. They were provided with saws for cutting through bone. The classes began with a closed circuit television demonstration of the day's dissection by one of the anatomy teachers, known as demonstrators. The groups then copied the master dissection as faithfully as possible on their own cadavers. For the first few weeks their untutored eyes found it difficult to match the mess of flesh and bone they had uncovered in their cadavers with the beautifully clear diagrams in the textbooks.

'It's important, before you begin to cut, to identify the bony landmarks underneath the flesh,' explained the demonstrator during the first session. She told students to feel the bones at the base of their own necks and upper chests, then, having found them on their cadavers, to dissect the area, including the breasts if they had female bodies. Each student had a turn, watched by other members of his or her group. 'Rub that bit out,' remarked a critical group member of an ugly cut. 'Too late,' came the rejoinder. 'My nose needs a rest,' announced one student, moving away from his table and the pungent odour of formalin.

'It's quite an experience – not as bad as I thought,' commented another. 'When you think you're actually cutting something that was one of us, then it gets to you a bit, but as long as you block out that it's a human being, then it's just like doing A Level dissections on rats – only just a bit bigger. I'm not looking forward to learning it, but doing it is good fun.'

Everyone seemed similarly enthusiastic. Sarah declared it 'brilliant' – easily the best thing she had done so far. 'It smells, but you get used to that. And it's a bit of a gooey mess – we wouldn't have recognised anything unless the teachers had pointed it out. But by the end of the year we shall have to know the structure of the whole body, including more than two hundred bones in detail.' Ese looked up from her dissection with shining eyes. 'The nerves are supposed to be white, elasticky things, and you can easily mistake them for fat or connective tissue, but when you actually find one, it's really good.' Dong Chiu, frowning with concentration as she dissected a breast, commented, 'It's quite exciting, but very slow. The skin is like shoe leather, very tough. I felt a bit squeamish when the demonstrator cut through the breast, because I could imagine that on me. But now I don't, which quite surprises me.'

When the dissection was over, students had to clean their cadavers up and sprinkle them using a watering can containing a solution of phenol to keep them supple and easy to cut in the weeks to come. If the bodies were allowed to dry out, they would become impossible to dissect.

After a few weeks, the dissection sessions became an event which most students, far from dreading, looked forward to. The Students' Union president, Marie-Louise Carden, explained why. 'Anatomy is a great social event because it is the only time in the week when the whole year is together in one room in a situation where they can wander round and chat to one another. It's the place where you find out who's going out with who and everything else that is going on at Mary's.'

Eight months later, when the dissection had been completed, every cadaver was reconstituted and buried, and a memorial service was held in memory of the individuals who had made the anatomy course possible. All the students were invited, but only a handful attended. Sarah Holdsworth was one of them and she found the experience very moving. 'It brought it home to me for the first time that my cadaver had been a real person.'

The dissection classes were complemented by a series of parallel lectures and vivas, designed to take students through the body bit by bit in minute anatomical detail. The vivas (short examinations in which students were questioned orally) provided invaluable experience for end of year exams and for their entire career at medical school, which would be dominated by oral exams. Every week students assembled in groups around 'their' cadaver for the dreaded anatomy viva. A member of staff sat at the head (literally) of the table and questioned each student in turn. Anatomy demanded a minute knowledge of bones, nerves and muscles throughout the body and the structures which connect them. Students were taken through the entire body during the course of the year. Prudent students spent several hours swotting up on the part of the body in question before their weekly grilling.

In their second term Mark, Nick, Sarah and Jane who were all in the same anatomy group nervously awaited the arrival of Dr Kerry Davies, who would question them on the previous week's dissection. 'Last week we began to look into the thigh,' he reminded his group, proceeding to question them in turn about the intricate network of nerves and blood vessels they had observed. The feats of memory demanded were considerable. Here is Dr Davies's first series of questions, addressed to Jane Morris.

Davies: 'Can you tell me something about the origin of the femoral artery?'

Jane: 'It's a continuation of the external iliac artery and it goes under the inguinal ligament to become the femoral.'

Davies: 'Where does the external iliac arise?'

Jane: 'From the common iliac, which fits into the internal iliac and the external iliac and that comes off the abdominal aorta.'

Davies: 'At about what level?'

Jane: 'L4.'

The questions continued, exploring the anatomy of the thigh

in minute detail for a remorseless thirty minutes, and woe betide anyone who answered less fluently than Jane. By tradition the viva was followed by an extended tea break which gave students a chance to lick their wounds and receive commiseration.

Physiology was another of the three subjects that loomed large during the first year at St Mary's. The course, consisting of lectures and practicals and tutorials, was designed to give students a good understanding of how every system in a normal, healthy body worked. The professor of physiology, Charles Michel, felt that his subject underpinned the whole of medicine. 'Unlike anatomy and modern biochemistry, it does not have much of an image among the general public. But it is the basis of rational thinking in clinical medicine and should foster problem-solving attitudes. It is also a subject in which they can learn to be critical. I am very anxious to encourage them to question what they read in textbooks and are told in lectures.'

The core of physiology teaching took place during the weekly practical sessions on Thursday afternoons, when students had to make observations about themselves or their colleagues and draw deductions from them. They were told that they would do lots of experiments on healthy young people – themselves, in fact – to measure things like respiration, urine production, bleeding time and response of muscles to electrical stimulation. In one particularly memorable early practical class, physiologist Dr Michael Rampling explained how to prepare a slide of blood and how to count the cells on the slide under a microscope.

'What you might have noticed,' he continued, 'is that there is no blood around on the bench for you to do any experiments on. So what we're going to get you to do is to take blood from one another, which is an important technique you should all be familiar with.' He introduced a senior colleague, Professor Sirs, on whom he proposed to demonstrate the technique of blood taking.

As the professor obligingly rolled up his sleeve, Dr Rampling demonstrated the equipment and outlined the pitfalls. 'The plunger in the syringe is a bit sticky, so you should push it backwards and forwards at the beginning to make sure you can move it around easily. It's obviously embarrassing if you find out that you can't move the syringe once you get the needle into the arm. The object of the exercise is to get in fairly quickly, because he will only feel anything while you penetrate the skin – once you've gone in, he won't feel any pain at all.'

Pale-faced students watched in dead silence as Rampling slid the needle into the professor's arm and pulled back the plunger, sucking the syringe full of crimson. The blood was put into tubes, each containing a few crystals of anti-coagulant to keep it liquid. Without that, the cells would quickly clump together, making the blood impossible to work with. He warned them that they should remember to wear gloves at all times when working with 'foreign blood' (i.e. blood that did not come from them) because of the risk of catching diseases such as Hepatitis B or AIDS.

Students then paired up to practise bloodletting. The victim rolled up his or her sleeve and a cuff was placed on the upper arm to force veins up towards the surface. The blood taker chose a fat vein, offered a silent prayer and pushed the needle in. An anxious student with trembling hands faced with an unwilling victim could make several attempts without drawing blood.

'You can't miss, they're standing up like cables,' commented Dr Rampling to a nervous female student. 'Now go in fairly smartly, along the line of the vein.' Once the samples had been obtained, each student took his or her own tube full of blood and began experimenting with it. There was intense concentration and low chatter throughout the laboratory as students prepared slides from the samples and examined the blood under microscopes in order to learn to recognise different types of cells and to calculate the number of white blood cells per millilitre of their own blood. It was an intricate procedure, especially hard for those students who had not taken biology A level and had no experience of microscopes.

Biochemistry – the chemistry of body processes – was the third pillar of the first-year curriculum and, as in anatomy and physiology, teaching took place in lectures and practicals. The laboratory sessions gave students the opportunity to do experiments with human and animal cells and to understand and carry out some of the standard biochemical tests performed in hospitals, which junior doctors order every day.

The biochemistry course was designed to give students a sound appreciation of the underlying molecular nature of health and disease at the cellular level. In his introductory lecture Professor Bob Williamson, like all three heads of department, stressed the great importance of his subject as a foundation of modern clinical medicine and told students that by the time they qualified, biochemical research would have produced exquisitely precise techniques for treating a whole host of conditions. He also pointed out that a glance at the papers in any current medical journal would underscore the importance of biochemistry in all branches of clinical research and practice.

'I like to think of this course as being a course in molecular medicine,' he told the students. 'I think we're trying to give you an understanding of the cellular and molecular processes that underlie the cases you're going to see when you begin to meet patients. A lot of what you will learn is underpinned by a knowledge of the way biochemicals, genes and cells work.'

The first year involved a lot of rote learning of enzyme pathways – the series of biochemical reactions which, for example, allow the body to take in food, drugs and gases and convert them both into substances useful to it and into unwanted by-products which can be expelled. During the second year the subject became more patient-oriented, as students learned to connect what was happening at a cellular level with particular diseases and their symptoms. Throughout the course students benefited from St Mary's status as a leading genetic research centre. They learned how to search for faulty sections of genetic material which gave rise to diseases and abnormalities, and were taught the rudiments of DNA analysis and gene cloning.

In January, just as the first years had settled into their academic routine, they found themselves facing their first set of exams, known as Sessionals. These took place every term and were a sort of dry run for the end of year exams, an opportunity for the new intakes to gauge the standard of work required and the amount of work they would need to do to meet it. Many students did extremely badly and realised for the first time what they had let themselves in for. Sarah Holdsworth, for example, got thirty-two per cent, which put her near the bottom of the year.

Respite and relaxation from the pressure and monotony of pre-clinical medicine came in March in the shape of Rag Week. This annual event was organised by a committee and almost all the students who took an active part in the proceedings came from the first and second years. Mark George was Rag Secretary during his second year and spent six weeks planning events, ordering beer and hiring cleaners. Every year, the Rag raised thousands of pounds for charity during a week of revelry that began with the Paddington Breakfast Party.

At seven o'clock on a dark, damp March morning, Paddington Station was invaded by scores of medical students and a jazz band. Fey Probst and a friend, both wearing flimsy pyjamas, were stopped by a member of the public as they passed the hospital's psychiatric wing. 'Do the doctors know you've got out?' they were asked. As sleepy commuters stepped onto the platforms, they were surrounded by grinning, over-exuberant medical students selling Rag Mags. They were clad either in pyjamas and dressing gowns or in surgical masks and gowns and their sole sales tactic was to cause persistent annoyance to commuters until they caved in. 'Would you like to buy a rag mag?' they shouted. 'Very good value. All for charity. Only 50p.' Some people got very cross, but many paid up and the collecting tins filled quickly.

In no time 3000 copies had been sold and additional supplies had to be fetched from the medical school. But there was a problem: these copies had been intended for circulation within the medical school and contained a four-page insert for home consumption only, so a team of students set to work ripping the middle section out. A student supervisor explained. 'The green pages contain slightly dirtier jokes than the rest of the mag. We put all those in the middle pages so that we can take them out and they won't offend the commuters on the day. We had complaints from some of them a few years back, so now we think it's better to put the hard stuff in the middle.'

The highlight of the morning for the bemused Paddington commuters was perhaps the porridge eating competition which took place in the centre of the station concourse. Teams of students took turns to ladle porridge from a plate into each other's mouths with plastic spoons held between their teeth. Two male students evolved a quicker method: they took turns to plunge their faces into the porridge and transfer it from mouth to mouth by means of a passionate kiss. They quickly became the centre of attention and students clambered on to tables to obtain a clear view of their endeavours, roaring encouragement like a rugby crowd. The whole episode was filmed, and a few weeks later the BBC received a desperate letter from one of the two students, pleading that the material should never be shown. Friends who had qualified as doctors advised him he would be unlikely to find a post as a house officer if he appeared in such an escapade on national television.

At nine o'clock the first years scampered back to the medical school for their scheduled lecture on pupillary reflexes given by Dr Kerry Davies. Dr Davies entered a lecture theatre packed with semi-hysterical students, many still wearing pyjamas and dressing gowns, to squeals and cheers. 'Settle down,' he began optimistically. 'I realise it's Rag Week, but we still have the work to get through.' During the ensuing chorus of boos, two students dressed like garden gnomes sidled up to him on the dais. He tried to continue, but his efforts to instruct his audience on the effects of light on the eye were sabotaged completely by the arrival of the Hit Squad of four Flanners.

Flanning was a Rag Week tradition at St Mary's. Students from all years could pay, anonymously, for the hit squad to attack individual students with 'custard pies'. This year's hit squad, dressed in surgical gowns and lurid masks, had already sprayed liberal amounts of shaving cream on to paper plates to make the pies. Now they entered the lecture theatre and advanced menacingly along the gangway. Students cowered as they stood over them in pairs, each one holding two plates. Fey Probst was one of the first victims: four plates of shaving foam were pressed firmly into her face, hair and neck as scores of students cheered. Fey managed to peer through the foam with a brave face. Another girl suffered a variant of straightforward flanning: the Pintogram. The Hit Squad poured her a pint of bitter, if she drank it she would be reprieved, if not, the flanners would attack. She declined the beer and was duly plastered. Minutes later a foam-spraying battle broke out as several students attacked those around them with aerosol cans. Everyone ran from the theatre.

Sarah Holdsworth was a member of one of the hit squads in her first year and her assignment was to attack final year students in the canteen. 'I was terrified, they were all great big rugby players and I thought they would kill me. I went in, flanned them and then ran for my life.' By the time she herself was a final year student, Sarah had reservations. 'Flanning can be very cruel, because it is done anonymously in front of everyone else. It must be terrible to be a victim if you don't have many friends. I don't really agree with it.'

The Scavenger Hunt was a popular Rag Week competition. The organisers made a list of exotic items which could be obtained somewhere in London, ranging from famous people (who had to be kidnapped) to trophies from famous places (which had to be stolen) and points were awarded for each. Players had to pay to enter and the winner was awarded a handsome prize. High points went to street signs for Harley St and rival London hospitals like Guy's, to porters' hats and silverware from West End hotels. Particularly good booty was auctioned off to raise further funds. 'The police always come and say it's all right, as long as you hand it back,' commented a veteran scavenger. 'Trouble is, it never is handed back, and so we get into lots of trouble.'

The toga party and slave auction were perhaps the most bizarre events of Rag Week. The former would have been a standard disco, but for the fact that all the participants came dressed in togas of varying degrees of brevity. These togas, crudely impro-vised from sheets, were also required dress for 'slaves', the first year volunteers who were were herded on to a stage to be sold for charity to the highest bidder. Ese and Sarah offered themselves. 'Some girls were sold for £40 each, but no one wanted to buy us,' said Sarah afterwards. 'Eventually a group of second-year boys bought the two of us and another girl as a job lot for £15, but it was very humiliating. Afterwards we realised that the secret was to wear a short toga – ours came right down to the ground.' Slaves were required to perform menial tasks such as cooking, washing up and cleaning. One group of purchasers required a posse of slaves to warm their respective beds.

What was the function of Rag Week in the life of the medical school? The Dean described it as 'that annual Dean's agony: the most worrying week of the year'. Every Spring he received phone calls and letters of complaint from outraged members of the public, most of them incensed by the racism, sexism and general tastelessness of the Rag Mag.

Every year a large number of students got extremely drunk and a sizeable minority were apprehended by the police. Certainly it provided students with an opportunity to throw off their heavy academic yoke for a few days and let off steam. (It also employed their considerable energy in a good cause: in 1987, for example, Mark George was delighted to have raised £8000 for blind children.) But its roots seem to go deeper: a hundred and fifty years ago dirty jokes and lewd rhymes were an established part of medical teaching and rowdy behaviour frequently brought lectures to a halt. Medical students of that period had an appalling reputation, and a doctor who was a student in the 1840s recalled that 'drinking, smoking and brawling were the occupations of the dissecting room. It was no uncommon thing to see a regular battle among the students, parts of the human body forming their weapons.'

The medical students of the 1980s were of the same species and used similar safety valves. Rag Week was one of them, an eruption of antisocial, atavistic behaviour among the pre-clinical students, now a tight-knit group, bound by rites of initiation and fear of trials to come. For those who stayed outside the group, life was a little lonely. Dong Chiu, for example, took no part in the Rag.

Secret societies were another facet of life at St Mary's. There were two exclusive male drinking clubs: the Gentleman's Club and the County Club. Mark George and Nick Hollings belonged to the latter, a club with only fifteen members who had all been recruited by invitation. Mark described its activities. 'We meet once a month at fine hostelries in London and the country. The members are either students or junior doctors. We have mixed evenings where we let women in very, very occasionally.' It was in response to such exclusively male associations that Jane Morris, Sarah Holdsworth and a group of second-year friends formed The Black Widows, a secret ladies' society. It started when they bought four first-year men at the Slave Auction in Freshers' Week and used them to prepare and serve (dressed in dinner jackets) a sumptuous dinner. This became an annual event.

The Rag Ball marked the end of Rag Week and the beginning of the exam season. The first years faced exams in anatomy, biochemistry, cell biology, histology, genetics, physiology and statistics. By now they had hundreds of pages of notes and a fat textbook for each subject which they had to learn. Ese's schedule was typical. 'I've been working for more than twelve weeks. There's no time for social life and nothing happens around the medical school because everyone feels too guilty. No one's in the bar. I set myself a timetable: get up at eight, breakfast at nine, sit down for an hour then have a break for ten minutes. Repeat that for the next three hours, have lunch, then do that again for three hours, have tea, then another few hours and I carry on till twelve or one, depending on how much I've got to do. I do that every day – if you have more than half a day off you feel so guilty. I haven't had any days off.'

Jane also revised for three months. 'It's just rote learning of pages and pages of notes – horrible. The more you know, the more there is to know. You get all the past papers and find out what comes up regularly and you learn as much as you can, about fifty or sixty essays.' One of their friends revealed that he was getting through two jars of instant coffee per week. 'It's expensive on Nescafé, but nothing else, because you don't leave your room.' Mark suffered an attack of panic two weeks before the exams when, as he put it, he 'cracked up'. 'I couldn't remember things that I'd revised only a few hours before and became convinced that I wasn't going to pass. However, I took that night and the following morning off and everything was fine after that.'

There was a lot of group revision as the exams drew nearer: students pooled knowledge and ideas as they cross-questioned one another, and the sessions broke the tedium of solitary revision. Ese and her friends swotted together in her bedsit in Nutford House: five girls sitting barefoot on the bed and floor or curled up in chairs, all cradling mugs of instant coffee as they pored over multiple choice questions. There was great good humour, affection and co-operation between the students. In the common room at Wilson House, Mark and four friends revised for their anatomy exam, answering questions with the help of bones drawn from a box. The preposterous abstruseness of some of the questions provoked near-hysteria. Eventually their enthusiasm for anatomy evaporated. 'How about a bit of gynaecological stuff? That's always good for a laugh,' suggested one of the men.

The written examinations began in mid-June. After students had sat the written papers, they faced the oral exams (or vivas). In most subjects only borderline candidates and those in the running for prizes had to sit vivas, but the anatomy viva was compulsory and terrifying. Two examiners took it in turns to grill candidates. Typically they would pick a bone and ask them to talk about it. Students would then be quizzed about the muscles originating near that bone, or the blood vessels. There were also limitless possibilities for questioning about the soft tissues. Many students felt they were fighting a battle which they couldn't win.

'The worst thing,' Sarah explained, 'is that they can just pick on anything in a viva, any little thing. And if you just don't happen to know anything about that particular thing, you can be in a lot of trouble and it looks as if you don't know anything.' Jane agreed. 'I've never been so frightened in my life. I was shaking.' Ese tried to work all night before her anatomy viva. 'I had never stayed up later than two o'clock in the morning, but I decided I was going to camp out with my books and bones. But I made it till about twelve and I went to bed. I was so nervous that I couldn't sleep anyway so I got up at five in the morning and the whole corridor was still scribbling away. Some students were feeling sick and shaking and I heard of some people who were physically sick. We suffered! And when it came to the exam, all the stuff that I had done at five o'clock in the morning was a total waste of time.'

In the dead time between sitting their last vivas and receiving their results, the students realised with a shock that summer had arrived. Sitting in sunny pub gardens, they contemplated their fate. Those who passed could look forward to three months off, those who failed would forfeit their summer holiday because the resits took place in September and they would need to revise thoroughly for them. There was a consensus that many people had done too little work. With the wisdom of hindsight, everyone agreed that they should have put in two to three hours a day right from the beginning.

On 27 June semi-hysterical groups of students clad in shorts and T-shirts jostled in the foyer of the medical school corridor awaiting their results. At last the Deputy Registrar of the Medical School emerged from the main office and pinned a notice on the results board in the main corridor. Terrified groups of students advanced gingerly towards it. There were two lists, one for those who had passed, the other for the failures – and it was immediately apparent that many had failed, a fifth of the year.

Sarah Holdsworth discovered that she was among them. She had never failed an exam before. After one look at the list, she burst into tears and ran out of the medical school. She stood on the steps outside, sobbing, 'I just can't believe I've failed.' Later, in the privacy of her room in Nutford House, Sarah howled with anguish, defeating her mother's attempts to comfort her. 'I was absolutely hysterical,' she admitted later. 'It was the biggest shock I had ever had in my life.'

Meanwhile in the bar, the successful candidates celebrated. 'It's a big relief,' grinned Mark George. 'I didn't work very hard during the first two terms and this term has been a bit of a nightmare, but I was lucky and it's come off.' 'I've passed as well,' confirmed Ese, 'but it's a terrible anticlimax – awful. You're supposed to be happy and jolly and jumping up and down, but you just can't be. Some of my friends failed and I just feel like crying for them. There's a disco tonight, but I just can't go to that: I'd be in tears.'

Eight of our students enjoyed a long summer holiday. Mark was typical. 'I'm going to enjoy as many social events as possible, starting with Henley, and then I'm off for two weeks to the Canaries. When I get back, I'll be working as an auxiliary nurse for a month to bring in some money and I might take the last week off to go to the South of France to get a suntan.' Most went abroad for a holiday and took a job at home, Jane and Ese both worked and took holidays abroad.

Sarah and Dong Chiu (who had not taken the first year exams because of illness) took a short holiday, then returned to St Mary's to revise for the resits.

Sarah had been devastated by the June results, but by the time of the resits she felt more confident. 'When I failed, the Dean said I wasn't a hopeless case, and he was sure I could pass if I got my act together. He told me to take at least three weeks off, then come back and go over it again. The staff have been really helpful; I've been taking essays down to them for marking. It was just my anatomy that pulled me down, so it was quite upsetting.

'It spoils your summer. I think the problem was that I didn't really know how to study. My A levels were physics and maths which are ninety per cent understanding, and chemistry, which you do have to learn for. But I'd never had to sit down and absolutely learn incredible amounts of information off by heart with hardly any understanding at all, like you have to do in anatomy.'

The resit results came out in the last week of September, just before the beginning of the new term. Again the candidates paced the entrance hall of the medical school, biting their lips and waiting for the lists to go up. Dong Chiu looked scared. Sarah sat head in hands, bleakly aware that this was her final chance: another failure would spell the end of her medical career.

The list was finally posted. 'Come on,' said Dong Chiu, patting Sarah's arm. Both walked slowly towards the board. Sarah saw her name in the list of passes, beamed at the paper and ran down the corridor, flushed with happiness, hugging everyone she met. Sarah later commented that failing her first-year exams was 'the best thing that ever happened to me – it taught me that I had to work.'

Dong Chiu failed at her first attempt and appeared a little upset but unsurprised. 'I got left behind because I didn't do A level biology and I had lots of problems with biochemistry and physiology and I didn't do any extra work, so I just got further and further behind. In the end, it was too much to catch up, so I just gave up. I realised I was slipping back when I came near the bottom in my sessionals. But it was too much to overcome, so I started thinking that I would like to do something else that is easier, like art. I felt very boxed in.' Now Dong Chiu would have to repeat the entire first year and take her resits in June of the following year.

The second year of the pre-clinical course brought new subjects in addition to the foundation disciplines of anatomy, physiology and biochemistry – and even harder work. As a compensation, students were given a tantalising glimpse of patients and there was a more clinical emphasis to the teaching. For example, in physiology, instead of learning how cells functioned, they studied whole systems like the heart. As before, the timetable consisted of lectures, practicals and tutorials.

The new second-year subjects were: pharmacology – the properties of drugs and the ways they behave in the body; psychology; sociology; pathology, the study of disease; statistics; and biometry – the application of statistics to biology.

Students now had to keep pace with some fourteen different subjects and found organising their time much more difficult. But the workload, though heavy, was more enjoyable, as Sarah explained. 'It is much more clinically oriented: we've been shown patients and had clinical demonstrations and little things we've been taught in lots of separate lectures have all slotted into place.'

Clinical demonstrations were particularly popular because they allowed students to see and participate in the process of diagnosis and to employ some of the basic scientific knowledge they had already acquired. A favourite clinical teacher was Dr David Thomas, who had won a place in the students' hearts during Freshers' Week with his spoof lecture. Now they encountered him in more serious vein when he presented two neurological patients to them in one of the lecture theatres in the main hospital.

'I hope this demonstration will make some of the things you are learning over the other side of the road in the medical school come to life and have some clinical relevance for you,' he said.

Students were asked to perform tests on the patients, both of whom had suffered damage to their nerves which impaired movement, and then, by using their knowledge of anatomy, to deduce where the damage had occurred.

Another popular lecturer was Dr Oscar Craig, who taught the

rudiments of radiology – how to take pictures of the inside of the body and which techniques were best suited to particular organs. In his final lecture, designed as rapid revision before the second-year exams, he whizzed through different types of imaging: CT scans, MRI scans and ultrasound scans. Then he changed tack, reminding students that their studies were about to enter a new phase.

'You're at such an important stage of medicine. Coming up to the end of the pre-clinical stage is exciting. Things change completely when you go over to the wards: real clinical contact begins then. You've heard me talk about technology, it's absolutely incredible and one is thrilled that it's gone this far. But are we as good at compassion, hand holding, care, as we were thirty years ago? I don't think we are. I want to say to you: go ahead with the technology. Move fast. But don't forget that the really important thing is your relationship with the patient. Care is what it's all about.'

These words elicited a long, warm round of applause from the students. But everyone in the audience was grimly aware of the fact that they would move on to the challenges of clinical medicine only if they cleared the next gigantic hurdle: the second-year exams. Revision was already well under way and was even more daunting than the previous year. Students had to spend hundreds of hours in the library with piles of books, writing and drawing endlessly in an attempt to commit thousands of words and hundreds of diagrams to memory.

Most of the country was suffering from election fever, speculating whether Margaret Thatcher would win a third term of office for the Conservatives. But at St Mary's all that mattered was revision. Mark and Nick worked together in their flat and Sarah joined them. It was more demanding but less mindless than first-year revision. Questions gave details of cases with the results of scientific tests which had been carried out and candidates had to work out their significance. It was a detective game whose players needed a good knowledge of physiology and biochemistry and anatomy and a firm grasp of practical procedures and how to perform them. The session was fun, but all three participants yawned repeatedly and looked very tired. They all admitted that it was a hard slog. 'After failing last year, I think I learned to work in a different way,' said Sarah. 'This term you have to knuckle down and forget about everything other than work. I'm not doing any sailing this term.' (Sarah had represented London University in international competitions and was captain of the Ladies Sailing Club. Her boyfriend was captain of the university men's club; they had met in her first year through the sport.)

'Spotting' was a widespread obsession. It involved scrutinising years of past papers in an attempt to spot patterns in the questions and predict what would come up in the next paper. In addition the medical school was rife with rumours about likely questions, which prompted frenzied last-minute revision.

Outside the sports hall at Wilson House the students milled around in the street before being admitted to the exam room. John Shephard admitted to feeling terrible. 'I don't know what has happened, there is mass hysteria. At midnight in the hall of residence, people are tired, fraught, there's only nine hours to go and things start getting out of proportion. We should know better!' Mark and Nick arrived together, looking drawn. Mark was smoking. 'I'm using it as a stimulant. This morning we've had anxiety states at the flat in Westbourne Terrace. I haven't slept.' A latecomer, purple with exertion, sprinted towards Wilson House entrance to be greeted by an irascible tutor yelling, 'Come *on*. We're waiting for you!'

Immediately after the last written exam everyone emerged into blazing sunshine and headed straight for an outdoor Pimm's Party which had been set up in the yard behind Wilson House. They laughed, cried, smoked, drank and compared notes on the last paper. It was a graphic display of the camaraderie of the group.

No one had liked the exam. 'It was horrendous,' shuddered Fey, 'one of the worst things I've ever done. Three out of the six questions were meaningless so I had no choice.' Mark agreed. 'Basically I thought it was a bastard and I'm pretty worried. I'm relieved they are over and I can relax before the vivas.' John said, 'It's the hardest work I've ever done, but the atmosphere here helps, everyone's studying and panicking and it motivates you. Also, I can't afford to fail and that drives me – even after two years. This weekend I shall go home, say hello to my wife and apologise for being such a swine for the past six weeks.'

After sitting five written papers in seven days the students had a few days to relax before the vivas began. There was a compulsory pharmacology viva but in other subjects around forty per cent of students faced a viva in at least one paper.

John Shephard went to see the professor of pharmacology, John Caldwell, for some last-minute advice on how to approach his pharmacology oral. The meeting turned into a coaching session on viva technique. Caldwell explained that John would face two examiners across a table and that they would question him for about ten minutes. 'Don't be too nervous and be prepared to talk,' he told him. 'Remember that, as long as you are talking, the examiner can't ask you a question you don't know the answer to. When something comes up that you don't know about, for heavens sake, say so. Don't dig yourself a pit and fall into it. It's important to bring the examiners to heel if you're asked something you don't understand or feel is inappropriate. You can do that once, but if you do it twice, you're in trouble.'

While nine of our students wrestled with the second-year exams, Dong Chiu was making her second attempt at the first year hurdle. It had been a difficult year, trying to get to know a new set of students and keeping on top of her work. 'When I started the first year again my main aim was to keep up and do everything I was assigned. I took lots of notes but didn't learn much so now I've got to get it into my head. I find the work dull when it comes in too large a lump. I felt left out in the beginning, but the second years have been very good – they looked after me. My family was very understanding. It cost them a lot for me to do this extra year, but they have been very good and haven't said anything to me.'

When the exams finally arrived, Dong Chiu found herself in a situation that every student dreads. 'I didn't realise they had revised the exam timetable and that the last paper was moved forward by two days. It was a combined paper on genetics, cell biology and histology, and I thought I had an extra two days to cover those subjects. So I was having a relaxing time after the last exam, when the phone rang and the tutor said there was an exam on and I had to rush down there immediately. So I was half an hour late, but I got extra time in the end. I have thought about what would happen if I failed again, but I haven't made any definite plans.' Dong's disaster happened because she was totally isolated from the rest of her year: everyone else knew about the change of timetable, but the news never reached her.

The first- and second-year exam results came out on the same day, 1 July 1987. The system for notifying results was different from the previous year: this time all students were to receive their results in an envelope, which they could either pick up directly from the main office of the medical school or have sent to their homes. Most students approved of the change, although Sarah Holdsworth, who had suffered a public failure the previous year, commented that, in the absence of a published list, those who failed would have to tell people the news themselves over and over again.

Inside the office secretaries sorted brown envelopes into alphabetical piles, ready for collection. Outside in the foyer, students waited for the summons. Jane and Sarah marched in together to collect their envelopes and tore them open in the foyer. Jane gasped with relief as she saw she had passed. Sarah was not only safely through, she was among the top ten students in the year. As they stood grinning at one another, Mark arrived and asked how they had done. He gave both of them a congratulatory hug before disappearing to fetch his own envelope with a grim 'Here we go.' Nick went in with him. They ripped open the envelopes in silence, then a tentative glance and mutual query – 'No probs?' – established the result and they flung their arms around each other's shoulders. 'Good man,' grinned Nick. 'Good news,' agreed Mark. They both reread the paper for the sheer pleasure of it, then headed for the bar. 'I think we deserve a drink.'

Ese, Will Liddell and David Copping had also passed. But there were nineteen failures, who in September would have to retake all the papers they had failed, before they could start clinical medicine, and Fey and John were among them. Fey had failed biochemistry. 'I obviously didn't do enough in the course of the year and I'm thankful to have passed four out of five,' she said on getting the result. John, who had also failed in biochemistry, was equally philosophical. 'Loss of neurones is the problem at my age, but I sensed it in the exam. I was quite relieved it was biochemistry because I can cope with that. I'll do another three weeks' work just before the resit. The great thing is that, if I pass that, they can't kick me out for another three years.'

After most of the other candidates had collected their results, Dong Chiu arrived for her envelope. She knew that, if she failed now, she would have to give up medicine. After the mistake with her timetable, she feared the worst. She ripped open the envelope and desperation suffused her face as she announced, 'I've passed everything except the last paper.' She bowed her head and began to cry. 'I don't know what's going to happen now.'

Five days later Dong Chiu was back at the medical school for an interview with the Dean that would seal her future: she was certain that the meeting would mark the end of her medical career. She sat outside his office looking sad and very lonely. The meeting was brief. He asked about her timetable blunder. 'You were given extra time, but it seems that you just went to pieces?' 'I was really in despair,' explained Dong Chiu.

'Well, you passed the other parts of the exam and the examiners were quite sure you didn't do yourself justice in the one you failed, and therefore we propose to make an exception and let you retake Section Three.' She smiled for the first time in days. 'What I want you to do first is to go home and have a good holiday. In September you have to pass if you are going to go on.'

Afterwards Dong said, 'I feel drained. I didn't know what to expect today. I shan't rest until I pass this exam. I'm going to have a rather dead time for the next few months.' In September, she passed and began her second year. John and Fey also passed their second year resits and started clinical medicine along with Will, Ese and David.

The remaining students, Nick, Mark, Jane and Sarah, had done well enough in their exams to take a year off from medicine to study for an intercalated bachelor of science degree. They could qualify for a BSc after just one year's study because their two years of pre-clinical science counted as two-thirds of the degree.

Sarah and Jane went to University College in the centre of London to study for a BSc in psychology. Nick stayed at St Mary's to study chemical pathology and Mark did physics with medical applications at Guys and the Middlesex medical schools. They all thought the BSc would stand them in good stead once they had qualified. Nick summed up their attitudes. 'I know people who aren't going to do a BSc because they feel as if they have been taking exams for ever. But a lot of people say that if you get a BSc you stand a better chance of getting a good job in hospital medicine.'

Sarah did so well in her second-year exams that she qualified for an MRC grant which helped pay her fees. Nick also got a grant, but Jane and Mark's additional fees were paid by their parents. (Students who were totally dependent on local authority grants to cover their living expenses found it difficult to finance a BSc.) All four found the BSc year stimulating and enjoyable, a welcome opportunity to read widely and think for themselves after the spoon feeding and rote learning of pre-clinical medicine. They also formed firm friendships with fellow undergraduates. They sat parts of the final exams taken by London University undergraduates after three years of study, and all performed well. Mark got a first and contributed to a published research paper, and the others received upper seconds. In the autumn of 1987, they received their degrees in a ceremony at the Albert Hall.

4

ON THE WARDS

It was the moment they had waited for: after the slog of academic science and the tyranny of exams, real medicine was about to begin. The pre-clinical course had encouraged familiarity with dead patients during the weekly dissection classes and occasionally offered tantalising glimpses of live ones in lectures. But despite the fact that students had spent two years in the shadow of St Mary's Hospital, as yet they knew virtually nothing of the actual practice of being a doctor.

Clinical medicine derived its name from the Latin word *clinicus* – person on a sick bed – and it concentrated on the study of patients and their illnesses; teaching took place in wards, outpatient clinics and operating theatres. Our ten students started the course in two groups. Fey, Will, Ese, David and John went straight on to the wards at the end of their pre-clinical studies in September 1987. The remaining five started a year later: Jane, Sarah, Nick and Mark had all completed BSc degrees and Dong Chiu had fallen back a year after failing her first-year exams.

A transformation in appearance accompanied the move from medical school to hospital. The standard undergraduate uniform of T-shirts and jeans suddenly gave way to the inoffensive professional dress associated with solicitors or teachers. And, to top it off there was the cloak of office: the clinical student's short white coat. Students had to buy their own white jackets and most purchased two or three from the Students' Union shop at St

Mary's during the first week of the course. Before setting foot in the wards, they also had to buy a stethoscope. John and Ese bought theirs from a medical instruments shop in the West End, which looked more like a museum, full of highly-polished wood and glass cabinets containing strangely shaped bits of metal. An old-fashioned shop-assistant displayed the considerable range available, and informed them that there were two different lengths to choose from: the 22-inch, which most doctors used, and the 28-inch. 'It all depends how close you want to get to your patients,' he commented. Both John and Ese opted for the longer version.

How would our ten students feel as they donned their coats and stethoscopes for the first time? Dr Oscar Craig had given them a preview of the moment during his stirring address in Freshers' Week. 'The day that you walk to your clinical course is a great day: you will be feeling fantastic. Chaps will hold their hands in their pockets, because that pushes the stethoscope a little further out of the pocket. And the girls will have them hanging round their necks, like necklaces – the most expensive and best necklace you've ever bought. You've worked for it, you deserve it and it's your badge of office. If you don't feel proud, you're in the wrong game.' These trappings of clinical studies dignified their wearers. Overnight, students turned into uniformed semi-professionals and began to sense the power they would wield as doctors. Most patients thought they were already qualified and pleaded timidly for information about their illnesses on the wards. Clinical medicine took the students into St Mary's and its local sister hospitals, which together served a population of 440 000, encompassing extremes of wealth and poverty. The elegant Georgian terraces of Bayswater fell within their catchment area as well as the 'bed and breakfast' hotels of Paddington and the tenements of North Kensington.

Most of the three clinical years would be based at St Mary's itself. The hospital was founded to serve Paddington, an area that grew from a small village to a teeming quarter of west London during the early eighteenth century thanks to the extension of the Grand Union Canal into the area, and the opening of Paddington Station. The original Norfolk Wing, opened in 1851, was designed by an architect who specialised in country houses, and it boasted graceful proportions, high ceilings and huge, elegant staircases seldom seen in a hospital. Many further buildings were added subsequently in less grandiose style, but the Norfolk Wing remained the main entrance to the hospital until 1988, when the Queen Mother opened a ten-storey block named after her. The Queen Elizabeth the Queen Mother Building was soon shortened to 'the new hospital', and the cluster of Edwardian and Victorian buildings on the opposite side of the road quickly became 'the old hospital'.

In 1987, when our first students started on the wards, they found St Mary's a place of astonishing contrasts. The new building was a spacious, gleaming palace of health care with wide corridors, small wards, pleasant clinic areas and stylish interior decoration. It contained the casualty department, eight operating theatres, several suites of research laboratories, lecture theatres, and beds for 300 patients. Next door was another recent addition: the Paterson Psychiatric Wing. The old hospital on the opposite side of the road was a labyrinth of corridors and bridges which connected the various wings. The wards were antiquated: large, high-ceilinged, echoing rooms with long rows of beds and minimal privacy for patients. Waiting rooms and consulting rooms were cramped and gloomy. Many of the buildings were too small, dark and inconvenient for the efficient practice of modern medicine.

Another focus for clinical teaching was St Charles's Hospital, off Ladbroke Grove in North Kensington, five kilometres from St Mary's. A small district general hospital, it had close links with the teaching hospital and many consultants worked at both places. St Charles's was built in 1881 as a paupers' hospital on the site of the Marylebone Workhouse. It was an attractive three-storey building of yellow and white brick with a tall water tower that towered over the network of terraces north of Notting Hill and dominated the landscape of Victorian west London. Though visibly poorer and much more cramped than St Mary's, St Charles's was extremely popular with doctors and medical students because of its human scale and friendly atmosphere. Many of the nurses had worked there for decades and were familiar with the problems faced by new medical students.

St Mary's, like many medical schools, introduced students to the wards with a week of nursing and a week of lectures on first aid, talking to patients and history-taking. During nursing week, each student worked the hours and undertook the duties of a nursing auxiliary, thus learning the routine of the ward. He or she also learned the importance for medical students and qualified doctors of establishing good working relationships with nursing colleagues, and especially the ward sister.

John Shephard and Ese Oshevire found themselves at St Charles's, where ward Sister Mary Rose Burke told them that she hoped they would understand the ward routine by the end of the week and realise the key role played by nurses: they were the patients' advocates, the patient-doctor intermediaries who watched over patients twenty-four hours a day. 'I also hope you'll find out a few of the things that irritate us. Little things like leaving notes around when you've been dealing with a patient instead of filing them away. Or leaving sharps around: if you take blood or give any other sort of injection, the needles often get left and somebody else has to pick them up, and you never know what type of patient it has come from, so you could actually pass on infectious diseases. It makes life easier for everybody if you clean up after yourself.'

Nursing week involved a great deal of wandering around looking lost. Students were given a tour of their ward and shown where linen, dressings, drugs and equipment were stored. They helped serve food to patients and watched doctors taking blood. 'Later in the week, we'll find some big fat veins for you to practise on,' commented one doctor to Ese and John. In the meantime, they learned to make beds with proper 'hospital corners'. They made tea and coffee for patients. They took their blood pressure – a procedure which suddenly seemed more complicated than it had been when they had taken one another's in physiology practicals – tested patients' urine, took their temperatures and dressed minor wounds. Most of all they talked to patients. Sister Burke felt that this last, which seemed the easiest task, was the most difficult. 'There is great skill in communicating with patients and it takes ages to learn. They come on to the ward after years at school and college and are expected to be able to talk to patients and they cannot do it. I think it is important that they see nurses who have gained those skills communicating with patients.'

Inevitably their ignorance of clinical medicine and inexperience often left students floundering in conversations at the bedside. Ese, for example, was kind and full of concerned interest. But when an elderly gentleman told her that he suffered from myeloma her response was a confused giggle. 'I'm only a medical student and I don't know what that is,' she explained. He replied patiently and without emotion, 'Myeloma is cancer of the blood cells,' and her face fell. It turned out that he also had a heart condition and had been in hospital many times before. Describing himself as 'a veteran in the field of medicine', he gave Ese some advice on how to treat patients. 'All patients really love you, but sometimes they are in pain and that brings the worst out in people. They don't mean to be aggressive, and after seventeen years, I know that. So as a doctor you've got to be caring at all times.'

For John, the demands of nursing week came as a shock after the academic routine of the clinical course. 'Up until now we have been in the classroom, academically orientated and very channelled. This blows the whole thing wide open. You have to take a different approach: you realise that you are here to work with people and that it's not just a question of science, which is all we've been fed so far. Coming here, you realise with a shock that the science is secondary and that the people are the main thing.' He was also stunned by the impact his white coat had on patients. 'It seems as though you suddenly assume the role of a person who can solve problems. A lot of patients ask you for information, or ask you to sort things out and you are expected to deal with this enormous system they have been pushed into, even though you are probably floundering just as much as they are.'

By the end of his week with the nurses, John sympathised with some of their criticisms of doctors' behaviour. He recalled an occasion when he and a nurse were in the middle of moving a patient and a doctor 'swanned in' and began examining him; he had also seen consultants leave a man undressed after a ward round. 'It is so undignified and unnecessary: we must always try to maintain patients' dignity. I hope I will remember and not make these mistakes, because it's people we're dealing with – they are not objects.'

Like their predecessors centuries ago, today's clinical students effectively become apprentices. But, whereas their forebears were attached to an experienced doctor for a period of years, contemporary students move from specialty to specialty, joining different teams of doctors for as little as a week at a time, and never more than three months. These teams are known as firms, and medical students are attached to them. They spend their first few weeks with medical and surgical firms, and must rapidly work out who's who in the hierarchy.

Firms differ in shape, size and organisation, but a typical one would be headed by one or two consultants (fully qualified physicians or surgeons) and would also contain a senior registrar (the pre-consultant grade) or a registrar, a senior house officer (a junior doctor who has completed at least two basic hospital jobs) and one or two house officers (the most junior members of the team: qualified doctors in their first supervised year of practical training who have just passed their final MB degree). Titles offer scope for further confusion in hospital medicine: all physicians and junior surgeons are addressed as 'Dr'. But surgeons who have passed all their postgraduate surgical exams (i.e. all consultants and senior registrars and most registrars), are known as 'Mr', a perverse professional relic of the days when physicians were medicine's university educated élite and looked down on the barber-surgeons, an unlettered tribe with low social standing. By the middle of the last century, surgeons had been admitted to the fold, but in England and Wales they clung to their old title (in Scotland most call themselves 'Dr') – and woe betide the rookie clinical student who addresses his surgical chief as 'doctor'.

The aim of clinical training is to involve students as thoroughly as possible in the work of the firm. This means sitting in on outpatient clinics and examining patients who have been referred to hospital by their GPs. They are allocated several patients on the wards, whom they are expected to examine, see daily and report back about to members of the firm. If the firm is surgical, they are part of the team in the operating theatre and take turns at performing minor tasks during operations.

Initially students learned mainly by 'clerking' their patients. This involved taking their medical history (asking the patients how they became ill and what symptoms they noticed), doing a full examination and noting down all the physical signs of their illness. For patients, this was a repetition of the grilling that they had undergone on admission to hospital, but most submitted with good humour. Students were also expected to monitor the patient's daily progress, and to note the treatment prescribed, any changes in symptoms and signs and the results of any tests that had been carried out. They also helped carry out the simpler routine tasks performed by qualified doctors. Students took it in turns to 'do the bloods' for the firm's overworked house officer. This involved getting in at 8 A.M. and obtaining a list of patients who required blood tests, then doing the rounds of the beds. Before they descended on patients, all students had to practise the technique on one another, but their first 'real' blood test was a nerve-racking experience nevertheless.

Ese's hands trembled uncontrollably as she took her first blood from a woman with 'difficult' veins which could not be seen. She was supervised by Dr Fiona Alexander, who advised the students always to confess their inexperience to patients before starting to take blood. Ese made three attempts before any blood appeared in the syringe and was so tense that she did not address a word to her patient until their mutual ordeal was over. When it was finished, she gasped, 'Goodness gracious, never again! I was in a worse state than the patient – I needed a stretcher afterwards. I feel terrible: sick and faint.' Indeed, Ese was so badly affected by the experience that she had to be sent home for the rest of the day to recover.

'You'll get used to it by the end of eight weeks,' commented Dr Alexander sagely. 'Most patients will have patience with you, If you can't get the blood the first time, they will let you have another one or two goes, but after that, I'd give up for their sakes.'

Medical students are neither qualified doctors, nor complete laymen, and their ambiguous status can sometimes lead to difficulties on the wards. Most firms lay down ground rules for students who are attached to them, as Will and Fey discovered when they joined the professorial surgical firm at St Mary's. On their first day the senior registrar, Mr Peter Rutter, showed them round the wards and briefed them about what they were allowed to say to patients. 'You must never ever tell a patient that they have cancer unless you have written proof that they have, and you must know whether the firm would like them to know. So if a patient asks you, you have to dodge that one and simply come back to us and say: "Does the patient know? Do the relatives want to know?" Patients will question you, but don't say anything off your own bat, because it is worrying if people are saying different things.'

Students were all allocated patients on the surgical firm and told to clerk them. During their week of introductory lectures, they had been issued with a long list of questions to ask during history-taking and many had also bought pocket books which promised to guide them through the maze of clerking. During the first few months they adhered slavishly to these lists and put every patient through the same interrogation, irrespective of his or her complaint. As a result, it was not uncommon for a new clinical student to take two hours to clerk one patient.

Will Liddell was sent to see an elderly man who was recovering from an operation to remove a tumour. He was receiving oxygen and wore a face mask. Will dealt with the problem impressively, patting the patient's hand to establish initial contact and then repeating his words to let him know that he had understood. He later admitted that he had found the visit difficult. 'It is tricky because he has cancer. I don't know exactly how much he knows himself and I have not been able to read his notes. It is difficult starting from my position of complete ignorance and yet being accepted as someone who should know what is going on.'

Will's very first ward round with the surgeons had reinforced his feeling that, after two years of pre-clinical study, he was only just beginning to learn some basic medicine. 'I don't think I'll ever forget the first patient that we examined. We all stood round, eight of us, and we were trying to extract a history and do an examination of the respiratory system, and the doctor asked us to name some causes of a cough – a cough being one of the most basic symptoms you could have. And we stood around thinking: "A cough ... maybe he has a cold?" And it struck me that we had been in medical school for two years and we could only come up with about two causes of a cough. I just felt completely at sea. The depth of my ignorance is astonishing, considering how long I've been studying medicine.'

Fey faced the toughest task of all the students on the firm since she had not only to clerk her patient, an elderly married woman, but also to present her findings to the Professor of Surgery, Hugh Dudley. She spent two hours with the patient in the afternoon asking about her current complaint, medical history and general health, then had to sit down with her thick set of notes in order to condense a complex seven-year medical history into a concise report ready for her presentation the following morning. She worked at the hospital until half past four in the morning, 'learning everything which could be known about that woman', then drove home across London. Her eldest son was already up, listening to a test match commentary. Fey abandoned all ideas of sleep and made him an early breakfast.

Professor Dudley was a surgeon of the old school. A stickler for accuracy, clarity and good behaviour, he was feared by students as one of the tartars of the medical school who could take people to pieces. The nine new students waited for him at the top of a large, echoing staircase in the old hospital, chatting nervously. Fey was frantically re-reading her patient's voluminous notes when the professor arrived. A grey-haired man in his mid sixties who wore a short-sleeved white coat and St Mary's tie, his first words to the students were, 'Welcome to the real world!'

He began by talking about life on the wards. He told them that they would face difficulties in 'tribalising' themselves into clinical medicine. 'I hope that over the next few weeks you will begin to feel at home in what will initially be a pretty strange environment. You have come here stuffed full of basic scientific knowledge, but you are about to enter a learning process which is much less formalised than the one you have so far undergone. There aren't textbooks to tell you how to do things, even though there are textbooks which tell you what to do, and you have to learn how to be comfortable with patients by actually doing it.'

Turning to Fey, he explained the purpose of her presentation. 'I am to lead you through a clinical encounter with a patient and

I want to see how we can develop a method of talking to and examining a patient. As we go I intend to undertake a critique of what you do. I am only using you as stalking horse, not as someone that I want to beat into the ground – although you will encounter plenty of clinicians who will do that during your undergraduate career.'

The students followed Professor Dudley crocodile fashion to the patient's bedside and he drew the curtains to create the illusion of privacy. Fey introduced the patient and began to outline her medical history, referring to her notes. Her patient had had a sub-total colectomy and a mucous fistula, she announced, and Professor Dudley invited the other students to decode the terms. 'You are going to have to learn a new vocabulary of technical jargon, perhaps twenty or thirty thousand new words, during the next three years,' he explained. The patient, a plump, game, elderly lady, smiled nervously.

Fey looked pale, tired and very tense. The professor started his questioning sweetly but ended up grilling them all. Asked to speculate as to what had caused the patient's problems, one student replied, 'There was some infection or something.' Dudley frowned and pounced. 'Don't say "something" – that's not a pathological term. Avoid conditional, hedging statements and try to be reasonably straightforward in your communication.' However, when Will Liddell tried a straightforward 'I don't know' in response to one question, the Professor said testily, 'Now look, I don't ask a question that I don't think you can give an answer to.'

Another student was chewing his fingers. 'Stop biting your nails,' barked the professor. 'You have *got* to professionalise yourselves. Would you like to be interviewed by a doctor who is in the middle of biting his nails? As far as your patients are concerned, you are on show all the time. Indeed, one part of being a good doctor is being able to act a part, and you have got to come up to your patients' expectations. These are that you're a good egg, omnipotent and able to solve their problems. Nailbiters do *not* carry that message.'

Fey acquitted herself well: the professor told her that if she had been taking her final exams, her performance would have earned her a pass. Afterwards she said it had not been as bad an ordeal as she had feared. 'As a student, he doesn't expect you to know everything, but I think perhaps I was lucky that I was the first person to present anything to him. I think I got off remarkably lightly.'

All the students allocated to surgical firms were quickly given a taste of life in the operating theatre. David Copping was attached to the firm of Mr David Rosin, like Professor Dudley one of the medical school's more colourful characters. He was generally popular with students, but had a reputation for impatience in the face of ignorance or incompetence. On his first day in theatre David headed for the surgeon's changing room where he swapped his ward clothes and white jacket for the standard uniform of the operating theatre: green tunic and trousers, clogs, hat made of dish-cloth material and a paper mask which covered his nose and mouth. Mr Rosin arrived, a sharp-suited, clean cut man in his forties with mischievous eyes. He introduced himself to David then disappeared to change.

First the anaesthetists introduced David to their technology and he watched as an elderly lady was rendered unconscious by a simple injection into the back of her hand. Then Mr Rosin taught him how to scrub up, the ritual cleansing that precedes all surgery. It's called scrubbing, but although the whole of the forearm is thoroughly washed with a bright pink anti-bacterial skin cleanser, only the hands and fingernails are actually scrubbed with a nail brush. Mr Rosin told David to scrub for at least five minutes. 'Scrub each finger in turn. It's the nails I am really worried about – that's where the dirt is.' Once the washing had been completed, David had to turn off the taps with his elbows and dry his hands and arms on a sterile towel. Then he was taught how to wriggle his way into a long green sterile gown and wait while the theatre sister tied it at the back. The final torture was donning his surgical gloves, an intricate manoeuvre in which the skin-tight sterile gloves had to be pulled on, then peeled back to cover the sleeves of the gown. 'Don't touch anything that isn't green from now on,' warned Mr Rosin as he led David into the theatre. The only green things in theatre were the sterile drapes covering the patient and the instrument trolley.

The operating theatre was a gleaming white room full of machines, instruments and shiny bits of metal, a bare, bright place without shadows. It was noisy: every sound seemed exaggerated, whether the bleep of a monitor, the clank of the ventilator or the splutter of the suction machine. The operation involved the patient's leg and Mr Rosin cross-questioned David about the anatomy of the blood vessels and nerves in that area. He was typically contemptuous of his replies. 'Your anatomy is atrocious. What have you been doing all these years before we let you loose on the wards?' David's sole practical contribution to a complex and highly technical operation was to hold a clamp.

After the operation, Mr Rosin took David into the cramped surgeon's tea room for a cup of tea. David confessed that, though he had not felt faint, he was 'worn out' as a result of standing on his feet for such a long period without moving around. Mr Rosin explained that, although surgeons often operated for hours at a stretch without feeling tired, their assistants rapidly became exhausted because they had little or nothing to do.

Some consultants were formal in their attitude to students, addressing them always as Mr or Miss; others were more relaxed, adopting Christian names from the first day. One of the consultant surgeons referred to them not as medical students, but as 'doctors in training'. She preferred them to introduce themselves as such to patients and told them never to give their first names – it sounded unprofessional. Behaviour towards patients was similarly varied: some consultants took pains to involve them in the ritual of bedside teaching, which could take more than an hour, others treated them as props, acknowledging their presence only at the beginning and end of sessions.

Occasionally students found themselves facing very seriously ill patients during their first days on the wards. David Copping's first patient was a fifty-nine-year-old father of three who had had part of his oesophagus (foodpipe) and all his stomach removed because of a tumour three years earlier. He was now back in hospital with a suspected recurrence of the cancer: he had great difficulty swallowing and had lost a stone in weight during the past month. He was unfailingly cheerful in the face of pain, discomfort and constant vomiting, but was clearly very anxious about his condition. David was good at talking to him and sympathetic to his problems, but like all new clinical students, he seemed uncertain how to deal with life-threatening illness. He coped by tending to underplay the seriousness of the situation, describing the patient's readmission as a 'minor complication' at one stage.

David had to present the case to Mr Rosin, who took the ward round like a *Doctor in the House* consultant. 'Incompetent twit!' he growled at a student who began a reply to his questioning with an 'Um'. David was picked up for stating baldly that the man had cancer. 'We tend not to use the word cancer around patients,' commented the consultant. 'We usually say "new growth" or "mitotic lesion". You have to be a bit careful.' He asked David to examine the patient in front of the rest of the group and emphasised certain rules. They should always conduct examinations from the patient's right side, in other words, leading with their right hands. A female student asked how left-handed doctors coped with this convention. 'It's a bit like playing golf: most professionals will tell you to learn to play right handed – it just makes life a lot easier. But if you are very left handed, you are better off examining from the other side.' When examining the abdomen, he told them, they should keep their eyes on the patient's face, so that they could pinpoint the site of any pain quickly and accurately.

Three days later David went to University College Hospital for an investigation into the cause of his patient's blocked oesophagus. Specialists passed an endoscope down the throat so that doctors could obtain a clear view of the obstruction. The endoscope worked like a tiny camera on the end of a long thin tube. The pictures it took were transmitted to a television screen in the corner of the examination room and David watched as it moved down the oesophagus. 'The raised, ulcerated tissue you can see there is all neoplasm,' commented the specialist, employing yet another of the euphemisms doctors use when discussing cancer in front of the patient. The tumour was almost completely blocking the patient's oesophagus and the only treatment possible was to

cut through it with a laser passed through the endoscope so that
the patient would be able to swallow more easily. A few days later
the man went home, but his cancer grew relentlessly and he died
two and a half months later.

Students attached to the same firm organised an on-take rota for
themselves, so that each in turn was given the opportunity to
shadow one of the house officers during a day and night while
the firm was handling all emergency admissions to the hospital
in its particular specialty. During these on-call periods, students
had their first taste of working with a bleep. They were issued
with a personal pager and summoned by doctors on the firm if
an interesting case was admitted. Full of novice enthusiasm, they
saw the bleeps as yet another badge of office and relished being
harnessed to their work.

Ese had a busy first day on take in the small, crowded casualty
department at St Charles's, where she was attached to the medical
firm. 'We're on take from nine o'clock in the morning right
through until the next morning,' she explained. Often Ese was
the first person from the firm to see emergency cases and was
expected to tell the houseman or senior house officer what she
thought was wrong with them.

An old lady she admitted had been found by her social worker
lying on the floor of her flat. She had had a stroke and had almost
lost the power of speech. Ese had to establish a system of hand
squeezing signals before they could begin to communicate; it then
became clear that the patient understood everything she said.
Later she saw a seventeen-year-old boy who was diagnosed as
having pneumonia. Ese was sent to explain his illness and treatment to his mother and sister.

'Everything we were taught during the pre-clinical course seems
relevant now,' she said. 'If only we could have had a little glimpse
then of what we would use it for, I might have learned a lot more.
We've actually already been taught a lot of the things they are
teaching us now but, because it was so boring, we didn't take any
notice – so we've got to learn it all over again. Everything is so
interesting now: you're using your hands, talking to people and
you don't have to sit down at a desk and flick through thick books.

It's like detective work.' She was surprised at how busy the doctors were, and how they often went without lunch and supper because of overwork. Another surprise was the amount of responsibility she had been given on the wards. 'You're expected to become confident in the space of a few weeks. In medical school you can hide behind a book, but here they notice if you don't turn up, and they heap so much responsibility on you and you've just got to take it.' As one of the few black medical students, Ese found that she elicited a particularly warm response from black patients. 'They are terrific. They treat me like their daughter and ask me where I'm from and always give me a specially big smile.'

John Shephard, like Ese, was on the medical firm at St Charles's, where his consultant was the Dean, Professor Peter Richards. Three weeks after the students had begun the clinical course, the Professor took them to see new patients, whom they had to examine and diagnose in front of the group. John began his examination in a rather unorthodox manner. He explained that he had forgotten his wristwatch and that he would have to time the patient's pulse rate with the help of an alarm clock which he extracted from the pocket of his white coat. Professor Richards appeared tolerant of this eccentricity, commenting, 'That's all right, provided that it doesn't go off.' The patient was weaker on his left side and John was asked to examine his nervous system by conducting a series of routine tests. He ran into problems because he could not remember the various nerve pathways and had forgotten how to test reflexes. 'I'm digging myself an enormous hole here!' he said despairingly. 'Anatomy! Anatomy!' Professor Richards replied. 'What have you spent two years learning?' But, as John put it afterwards, 'When the consultant is staring at you with his beady eyes waiting for an answer, it's very difficult to say, "I'm sorry, I don't know."'

John, like all the new students, was starting to learn the skills of palpation: feeling the patient's body with the fingertips in order to determine whether organs were the right size, in the right place and trying to detect any abnormalities. They were also learning to distinguish between the sounds they heard through their stethoscopes from the lungs, heart and abdomen.

Examination was a skill that students learned slowly and labori-

ously. John admitted he was embarrassed when he had to go up
to a patient and say, 'Look, I'm sorry, I know there's no need to
examine you, but I must learn.' And he described how students
performed their examinations awkwardly with a book in one
hand and had to explain to patients that they would have to
keep referring to the book because they had not yet learned the
techniques by heart. 'Most patients are very tolerant and put up
with us pushing and prodding them. I think they like to feel that
they are helping us learn.'

Over breaks in the canteen the students compared notes. They
found they were all left to themselves to hunt patients down to
clerk and examine. It was up to them to make as much of the
opportunity as possible. Having worked for ten years before
entering medicine, John particularly relished doing a job again.
'Two years out at medical school was good fun, but coming back
here, I realised just how much I missed working. It's particularly
nice on take in the evenings, when you actually feel you are
contributing something at last. I love having the responsibility.'

Far from relishing the lack of structure in the clinical course,
Dong Chiu, who was based at St Charles's for her first firm, found
it baffling and exhausting. 'I am not comfortable with the fact
that it is up to me to grab bits of knowledge here and there,
because I can miss a lot without realising,' she said. Dong admitted
that when she had first worn her white coat (she made it herself,
because she didn't like the cut of the bought ones) she felt like a
doctor, but very soon abandoned the fantasy. 'During my first
two weeks on the ward, I've come crashing down because there
is so much I don't know. Some people have managed to get to
every corner of the hospital to see patients and I have yet to do
that. We each get a handful of patients and mine are rather
difficult to deal with.'

Dong said that patients reacted to her foreign appearance and
accent in one of two ways. Most went out of their way to be
pleasant, but a minority disliked her and refused to talk to her.
Dong's English was excellent but her accent could create a barrier.
'Sometimes, when we are working in pairs and I am with a
student who is British-looking and speaks fluent English, I notice
that the patients warm up towards the other person a great deal

faster than they do to me. I have great trouble understanding people who come from the north or have strong Irish accents. I panic sometimes, which doesn't help.'

Ese had her first taste of life in the operating theatre when she spent her first night on call with a surgical firm at the Central Middlesex Hospital. The first case was an elderly man, admitted in agony because of a perforated duodenal ulcer which required emergency repair. The second was a classic surgical emergency: a seventy-seven year old man with an aortic aneurysm (a blood-filled bulge in the main artery carrying blood out of his heart) which was on the point of bursting. In the event of such a burst, the patient would bleed to death and so a major, four-hour operation was needed to repair the artery. The consultant surgeon was summoned from home to perform it, clamping off the over-stretched section of the artery, then replacing the weakened part with a plastic graft. Ese was asked to hold the suction apparatus which removed blood and other fluids. Afterwards she was exhausted and said, 'It's very interesting, but I couldn't do it. If I think about all the hard work I'd have to do before I got to that stage, it's just too much. Hospital medicine is so hectic and the hours are awful. I don't think I could do it for more than three or four years. I think I'll be a GP.' It was half-past midnight and Ese confessed that all she wanted to do was have some food and go to bed. Unfortunately there were still some more patients to look at in casualty.

Will Liddell, who was also on take in casualty at Central Middlesex with a medical firm, having completed his six weeks of surgery at St Mary's, heard about Ese's busy night with envy. 'At Mary's you'd have to be on the surgical unit for about three months to see all that,' he commented. 'There are no patients there because of the cuts – they can't afford to operate. I went into theatre four or five times the whole time I was there.' Will was helping to deal with a twenty-year-old man who had been brought in unconscious after an afternoon of heavy drinking. When he came round he was unable to give any useful information to the doctors and began vomiting copiously everywhere. After an extensive mopping-up operation, Will was asked to assess the patient, a difficult task since every time he attempted to take his blood pressure, the man fought him off, convinced he was being given an injection.

Another venue for medical student teaching was the out-patient clinic, where students could interview and examine scores of patients in a single morning or afternoon. Sarah Holdsworth found herself in the busy out-patient department of the Central Middlesex Hospital where she was attached to the surgical firm of Mr Michael Henry, a consultant with a dry sense of humour. 'A lack of imagination,' he said at one stage, 'is a distinct advantage for those embarking on a medical training.'

Mr Henry, who was also the clinical tutor, said his main aim in teaching new clinical students was to get them to adopt a humane approach to patients. No one expected them to come up with a diagnosis or demonstrate familiarity with the physical signs of diseases, but they could play an important role by talking to and supporting the patients. 'They are actually doing a highly responsible job now – because we need their help. We may ask them to take blood and organise blood supplies for a patient's major operation the following day, and if they put the blood in the wrong bottle, that patient will have a mismatch and the consequences may be dire. They have to suddenly come to terms with the fact that life is rather serious and they have to adopt very different attitudes. They have to come into the hospital at eight o'clock in the morning – which comes as a shock to some of them – and they may have to work until late into the night.'

On her first morning in out-patients, Sarah saw many patients and had to abbreviate the interview technique she was learning to use on the wards. After taking her into several consultations with him, Mr Henry told her that the first patient he wanted her to see on her own was a young woman with a breast lump who had just been referred to him by her GP. She would have only ten minutes to spend with the patient and must therefore restrict herself to just a few questions. 'Remember this patient is only twenty-one,' he told Sarah as he propelled her towards the lion's den. 'She is going to be dreadfully anxious and I rely on you to make her feel as comfortable as you can. Get her confidence.'

White-faced and uncertain, Sarah clearly felt only marginally less distressed than her patient as she entered the consulting room.

'Hi, I'm Sarah,' she said, her voice husky with nervousness. The girl, equally pale, told her how she had discovered the lump in her breast a month earlier. Sarah began taking a history but very soon ground to a halt. 'I've run out of questions,' she confessed. When Mr Henry arrived, he showed Sarah how to examine the woman's breasts, but, to everyone's relief, the lump had now disappeared.

Sarah enjoyed her morning in the clinic. 'There's a lot of pressure in out-patients, and Mr Henry puts you on the spot, but that's the best way to learn.' Sarah had now forgotten most of the facts that she had learned on the pre-clinical course, and according to Mr Henry, she was typical. 'When I try to ask for certain information which they should have culled during the pre-clinical course, it is very rare to get any response at all. I am sure the pre-clinical staff would be horrified by this, but I think that most students see the pre-clinical course as a route that they have to take in order to come into clinical medicine.' In his view an integrated course of the kind already in operation at some other medical schools was inevitable and essential. 'At the moment, because of the compartmentalisation, students cannot see the relevance of some of the things they learn in their first two years – and that is a tragedy.'

Will Liddell, for one, agreed with him. 'The pre-clinical is a very poor preparation for training as a doctor,' he said. 'I would have preferred an integrated course: at the moment the course is trying to teach academic skills and provide an apprenticeship, but it actually falls between two stools and fails to do either adequately.'

However, Jane Morris, also with a surgical firm, but based at St Mary's, said later that she was grateful for the knowledge she had acquired during the pre-clinical years and was glad to have done a traditional curriculum, as opposed to one where students began clinical studies alongside basic sciences in the first year of the course. 'I feel very new as it is, having to go to see patients, even after two years at medical school. I feel I don't know enough. In my first year, when I knew nothing about the human body, I would certainly not have been ready to see patients: I think I would have felt completely stuck. As it is, although I don't remember all my anatomy, at least I have a vague idea about the structure of the body and how it works which I can build on.'

The Dean was well aware of the criticisms but his views were firm. 'I do not believe in introducing students to patients from day one. In terms of clinical skills it requires an enormous amount of time, concentration and effort – and that cannot be managed early in the course. But I would like to see them going into patients' homes to establish the social context of medicine from the beginning.'

He was also planning other changes. 'Everyone agrees that the course as a whole is too loaded with factual information and does too little to develop the intellects of students. For this reason we plan to reform the whole curriculum with a view to exciting and interesting students. We want to enable them to study in depth matters that interest them while retaining a core curriculum of things they must know.'

The first major change was planned for 1993, when a social medicine course lasting half a year would be introduced. The course would encompass psychiatry, general practice, geriatrics, community medicine, oncology, venereology and dermatology and much of the teaching would take place in the community.

For most of our students – no matter how well or badly they remembered their pre-clinical course – the first experience of life on the wards was an exhilarating one. The difficulties and embarrassments on the whole were outweighed by the sheer thrill of hands-on medicine. As Sarah put it, 'So far I have been very fortunate: the patients I have been attached to have all recovered and been sent home. It's been a success story. I think I have been fairly sheltered. The bad news is still to come.'

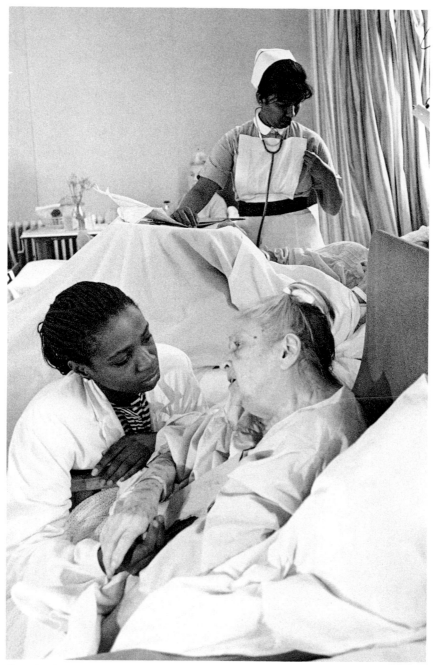

Developing a bedside manner: third-year student Ese Oshevire visits an elderly stroke victim whom she first met as an emergency admission in casualty.

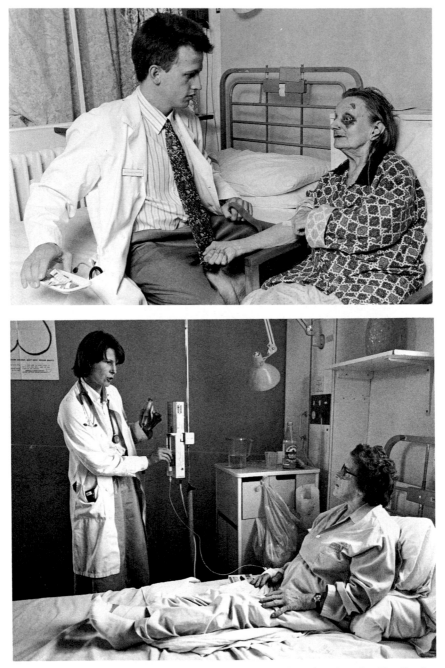

Doctors at last: after five years' training David Copping (top), *Fey Probst* (above) *and Sarah Holdsworth* (opposite) *finally begin treating their own patients on the wards.*

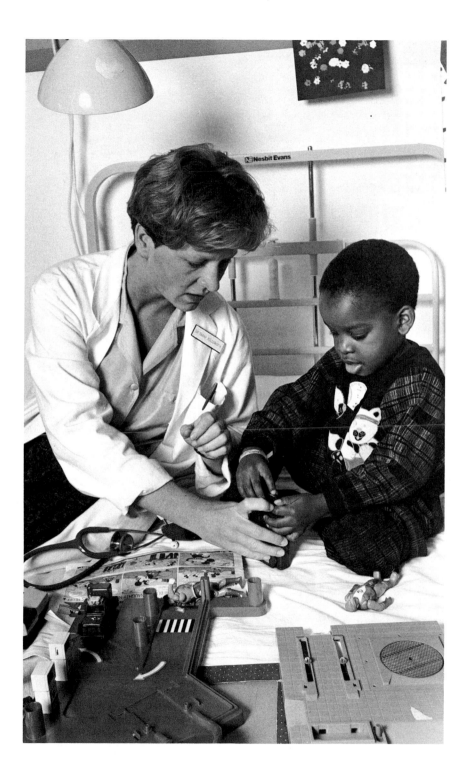

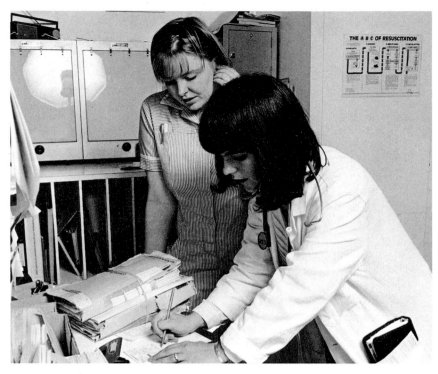

Jane Morris, whose first job after qualifying was as a surgical officer at St Charles's, divided her time between ward work (above), *and assisting at operations in the theatre* (below).

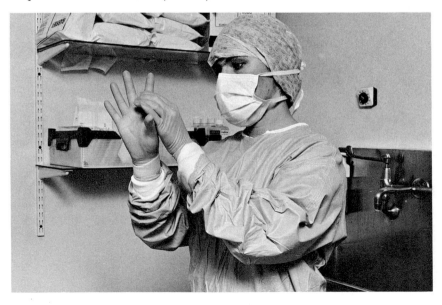

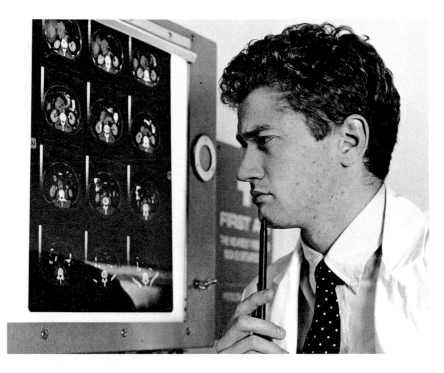

*House officers work long hours and shoulder considerable responsibility.
Above Nick Hollings checks a patient's CT scan. Below From left,
Sarah Holdsworth, Dong Ching Chiu and Mark George snatch a few
minutes for lunch in the staff canteen at St Mary's during their first jobs.*

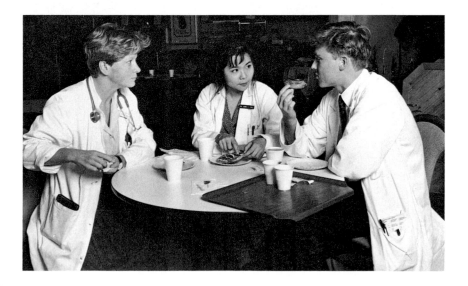

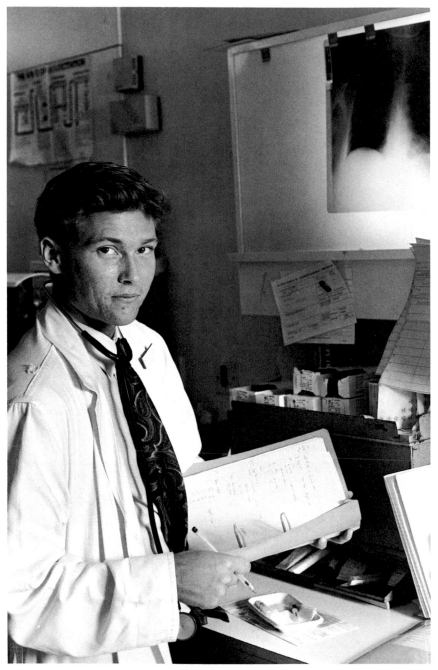

Mark George (above) *and Ese Oshevire* (opposite) *soon after qualifying. House officers spend hours filling in forms, searching for X rays and taking blood samples.*

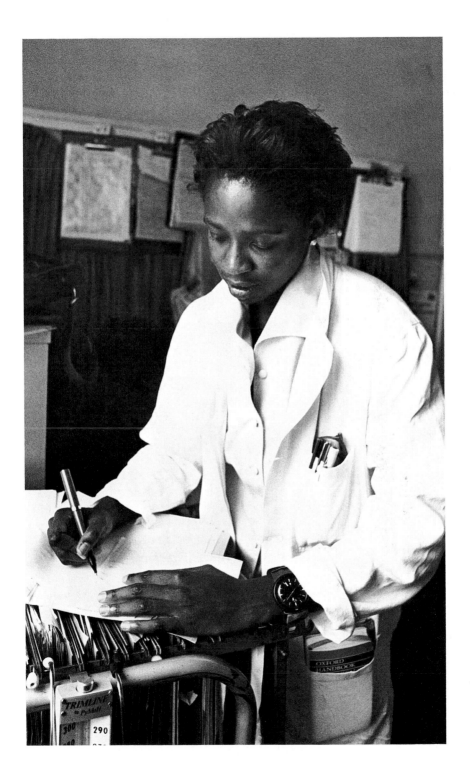

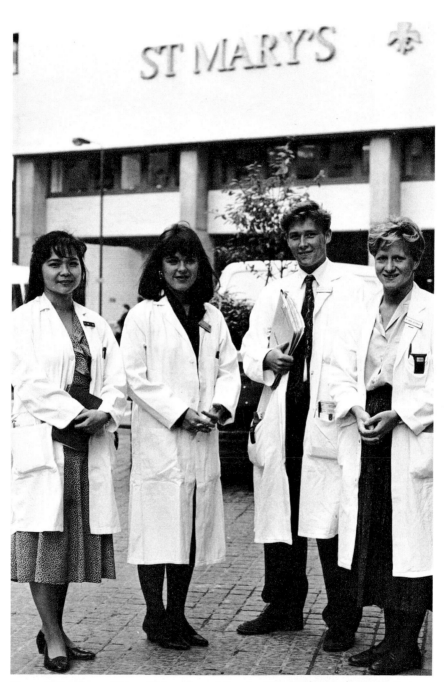

From left, Dong Ching Chiu, Jane Morris, Mark George and Sarah Holdsworth outside St Mary's new wing during their first house jobs.

—5—

TAKING THE STRAIN

After the first few heady weeks on the wards, students embarked upon the slow transformation from membership of the public to membership of the medical profession. The process of change had begun during their pre-clinical years in anatomy dissections, clinical demonstrations and conversations with their seniors in the medical school, but the key stages of the metamorphosis would happen now, as they progressed through different specialties, enlarging their knowledge of disease and honing their diagnostic skills. They were now beginning to think of themselves as doctors rather than students, but they were still ugly ducklings, often flapping their wings in panic, rather than confident professional swans. Ahead of them were the perils of childbirth, serious injury, abortion, death, the great traumas of life which in the twentieth century are kept out of public view. In dealing with these, they would have to learn about themselves and think hard about their careers.

The clinical years were both absorbing and demanding. Starting at an average age of twenty-one, students had to learn to ask patients intimate questions about their bodily functions, to deal with anger and grief, and to perform difficult procedures under pressure. The clinical course would take them into the labour ward and the hospice, would expect them to treat emergencies in Casualty and to field desperate questions from seriously ill patients. During three years they had to experience and assimilate the kinds of events and traumas that most of us take a lifetime to come to terms with.

They paid a price for this. In the final year of her clinical course, Sarah Holdsworth commented on its effects. 'You feel that you've touched on everything that was ever held private or sacred and nothing is sacred any more. The human body loses any mystique it ever had.'

At St Mary's the clinical course was divided into blocks, each lasting several weeks. After their initial attachments to medical and surgical firms, students spent fifteen months studying a range of major specialties: obstetrics and gynaecology, psychiatry, neurology, general practice, casualty, community medicine, orthopaedics and paediatrics. Each specialty offered a small number of lectures and seminars, but most of the time was spent with firms on the wards and in out-patient clinics. Halfway through their clinical course the students went back to full-time lectures and practicals during ten gruelling weeks of pathology – the study of disease processes – which gave them a working knowledge of the role of pathologists in diagnosis. At the end of the course they faced a major exam in pathology which counted as the fourth part of their medical degree. Then it was back to the wards and clinics for more medical and surgical firms, followed by a range of minor specialties: ophthalmology, rheumatology, cardiology, dermatology, ENT (disorders of the ear, nose and throat) and venereology.

Most learning took place while doing the job, as it had for centuries, and scarcely any time was allotted to reflection about the extraordinary things which students were seeing and doing. Even the most routine task, such as taking a medical history from an in-patient, could land a student in deep water, as John Shephard discovered during his first month on the wards. 'You can be asking a patient a specific question such as "Tell me why you are here," and you get something completely different that you don't know how to deal with,' explained John. 'You push on and try to get to the organic side of things, but the patient doesn't want to. He or she wants to talk about the other, more emotional side – and you just don't know what to do. You can't say, "I'm sorry, I just want to find out about your disease," because it's rude, and this may be the first time they've opened the floodgates.

You then have to go away and decide: Do I tell somebody? Is this in confidence? What do I do?'

Traditionally, students had been expected to evolve a competent 'bedside manner' simply by watching qualified doctors and copying them; there was no attempt to impart the skill of talking and listening to a patient as a formal part of teaching in medicine and surgery. However, in 1987 psychologist Dr Chris McManus and a group of young doctors at St Mary's launched a pilot scheme, using video cameras, designed to help new clinical students learn about interacting with patients.

Students were invited in groups of three to attend a session in which actors played various 'difficult' patients who had been admitted to hospital as emergencies and had to be interviewed by medical students. The consultations were filmed and then discussed by the three students, two observing clinicians and the actor-patients.

The seminars were controversial because some clinicians at St Mary's were convinced that communication could not be taught: students were either good or bad at talking to patients. Chris McManus was more optimistic: one could always improve by training. He felt that the general public had a right to expect that such skills would be taught in medical schools. 'It's assumed that if you are a bright, intelligent person with lots of knowledge who has seen lots of patients, then you're good at communicating. Unfortunately, it doesn't quite work that way.'

He explained why the seminars revolved around actors rather than real patients. 'With actors, we can control the situation. Just as pilots train on flight simulators, we can simulate a consultation for the students that pushes them to the limits. We can open up a situation that is normally very intimate and never becomes public because of the sanctity of the doctor-patient relationship.'

Most students were nervous at the beginning of the sessions and felt under pressure because they knew that the consultations were designed to make life difficult for them. When Mark George, Nick Hollings and Jane Morris attended one of the seminars in early 1989 all three were wary of what might lie in store. The session was led by Chris McManus and a physician from St Mary's, Dr Fiona Moss. Each student was allocated a difficult patient and they took turns to interview them for ten minutes in order to find out what was wrong with them. Jane Morris saw a hypochondriacal middle-aged man with chest pains who talked non-stop, and she was hard-pressed to get a word in edgeways. In contrast, Nick had to contend with a taciturn Welsh sheep farmer whose stoic underplaying of his symptoms masked serious disease. But the medical student's nightmare patient fell to Mark George. Chris McManus asked him to go to see 'Mrs Storey' who had been admitted the previous evening for investigation. While the others stayed in the seminar room watching the consultation on a video monitor, Mark went to a consulting room next door.

He found a thin pale woman draped in a hospital dressing gown sitting with arms folded. She stared stonily at the ground as Mark introduced himself and began to run through the standard history-taking questions. She had been admitted to hospital after coughing up blood, she told him. Blood tests had been taken and she was worried. No one had been to see her, nothing had been explained and she did not have time to sit around waiting. She was a successful marketing executive who should have been on a plane to New York, not surrounded by incompetents in Paddington. She wanted to see someone who knew what he was talking about.

Mrs Storey quickly lost confidence in Mark as he failed to answer her queries and, as she grew more aggressive, he became more nervous. A faltering question about the state of her marriage: 'How are things between you and your husband?' was the final straw, prompting a snarled, 'Is that really any of your business?' Mark, pale-faced and increasingly uncomfortable, eventually ran out of questions. In the adjacent observation room Jane Morris and Nick Hollings were glued to the video monitor, grimacing at one another as they watched Mark's mauling.

After ten minutes Mark's agony ended with a knock on the door and he returned to the seminar room visibly shaken. He joined the circle of observers and slumped into an armchair. Drs McManus and Moss began to assess his performance, using highlights from the tape.

The actress playing Mrs Storey joined the discussion, apologising to Mark for the hard time her alter ego had given him. Dr

Moss pointed out that Mark had forgotten to ask her whether she smoked – which she did – a serious omission when taking a history from a patient with a chest problem. Mark was also pulled up for saying that he would 'get things moving' in response to Mrs Storey's complaint that she had not been told the results of her tests, since as a medical student he had no power to authorise such action – a common trap, as Chris McManus recognised. 'There is a continual tension in the role of a medical student. You are slowly moving from being an ignorant member of the public to being a member of the clan with all the inside information, and you're halfway there, which is always a dangerous position to be in.'

Mrs Storey, he said, was a difficult patient but not unrepresentative. 'When people are ill, they often become miserable, depressed and hostile, and we cannot have doctors who can only deal with people who are fit, nice and happy. Mrs Storey is sick, needs help and the student has to cope with that.' Sometimes an encounter ended in confrontation. 'Students normally repress it: they pretend it hasn't happened and remember only the good patients they have seen. In these sessions we allow them to talk about the bad experiences so that next time they can handle them better. The social pressures on doctors and medical students are such that you tend not to admit your mistakes to your colleagues, because to do so is somehow to imply that you are not a good doctor.'

All three students said they had learned from the course – the the first communications training they had ever received. Mark commented, 'We've had all the guidelines on which questions to ask, but we are not normally assessed on how we talk to patients.' Jane agreed. 'Usually you go behind a curtain to see a patient, nobody knows what you are saying and, even if you make a complete mess of it, no one will ever know, so long as you get all the facts out in the end.' So far, none of the three had ever encountered a patient like Mrs Storey, but Jane had been told to go away by patients because she was a student. All three had been asked 'awkward questions' by patients about their illnesses. Have I got cancer? What's wrong with me? What do you think my chances are? What could go wrong in the operation? They had found that the only possible response was to be reassuring but non-committal.

Mark described how, when he was with a gynaecology firm, the doctor he was shadowing had asked him to wait outside while he visited a woman who was having a miscarriage. The students suggested that perhaps he had not wanted to be observed in case he got into difficulties and Chris McManus commented, 'There are many doctors who feel very worried about these things throughout their careers. They use all sorts of tricks to put off the moment of going to see the patient and, when they become senior enough, they send a more junior doctor in to do it.'

There were particular communication problems when students came into contact with disturbed or demented patients in the departments of psychiatry and geriatric medicine. Dong Chiu, whose first firm was medicine for the elderly, had an early encounter with a man who suffered from senile dementia which greatly disturbed her. 'I managed to talk to him quite well and I didn't think he was demented at all,' she later recalled. 'But people said he was – right in front of him within hearing distance – and he cried, which really upset me. When the others went, he turned to me and said: "You're not like them." So I stood there and kept quiet and I thought he understood.' Unfortunately Dong then found herself with a problem she was unable to deal with, 'He just latched onto me and followed me around, all over the place. And in the end I just couldn't cope with it, so I simply ignored him like the others, and eventually he went away. It was a very bad way of handling it.'

Dong was extremely depressed by the plight of many of the geriatric patients she saw during her first few weeks, but she knew she would have to adopt new attitudes. 'I have to learn to control myself, to realise that this is work and not let it affect me emotionally. We get some guidance from the course about how to take things step by step, which helps you get the work done, but it doesn't help you to stop feeling.'

Six months later, Dong Chiu felt that she had begun to deal with the problem. 'It's a matter of experience and learning that the world is not as pleasant a place as one had always thought. I cried a lot at first, but I wouldn't sit down and cry at a particularly sad case now. I've changed.' She felt she had become a harder person, but thought that was probably inevitable and necessary: doctors had to be emotionally tough in order to get on with their work.

She felt that hospitals stripped people of their individuality and humanity. 'It is such a professional relationship between doctors and patients: people in hospital are not given enough love. They are human beings, but in a hospital they don't seem human any more. I feel myself going that way as well – as if patients were a separate thing from persons.' She said that a week spent at a general practice in rural Berkshire had come as a revelation because she had frequently bumped into patients in the town, something which rarely happened in Paddington. 'It's a shock to recognise a patient out walking on the street, because he looks like a human being then, rather than a patient.'

Most of clinical medicine involved tagging along behind qualified doctors on the wards and sitting as mute observers in clinics, so specialties which offered students a slice of the action were automatically popular, although they often demanded reserves of courage and confidence. Childbirth was one of the highlights of the clinical course. Students spent six weeks learning obstetrics and delivered their first babies at St Mary's, then went out to a busy maternity unit for a fortnight in order to gain more experience. All students had to perform several deliveries before qualifying as doctors. The labour ward offered them a rare opportunity to play an important role in the medical process, but it also demanded a considerable degree of confidence and maturity. Suddenly, students were expected to take command of an emotionally charged situation and to guide women they had never met before through the uncharted territory of childbirth.

In a bare white labour room at Queen Charlotte's Hospital in west London twenty-two-year-old Nick Hollings found himself faced with the task of helping first-time mother Yolanta Tarnowska, who was only two years older than him, through the final stages of her labour. Nick began hesitantly, under the guidance of an experienced midwife, but gained confidence as he talked Yolanta through her contractions. 'Big push now. Keep pushing for me, right down into your bottom. Well done.' After a while the midwife let Nick take over the management of the labour, telling Yolanta to get used to his voice and do what he told her. By now, Nick was into his stride. 'Don't get confused,' he told Yolanta. 'Just listen to me, and let's push this baby out. Big push for me now, Yolanta. Excellent – I can see the baby's head!' A few minutes later, Nick eased the head out, then lifted the baby on to Yolanta's tummy and told her that she had a girl. 'Excellent,' he said, with typical lack of effusiveness, but a broad grin indicated his pleasure at the successful outcome of Yolanta's labour.

This was Nick's fourth delivery, and he now felt confident, but he admitted that the first time had been difficult. 'You feel very gauche walking up to a person you've never met before and saying, at a very intimate point, "Come on push this baby out, really try hard." But after you've done it a couple of times, you realise that they are there to give birth to a baby and if you give them a bit of encouragement, it will make it easier for them and quicker.' When the women were in pain during labour, Nick found his role more difficult. 'You don't really know where to put yourself. You feel very involved and you think: what can I do to make her feel less pain? In fact, the first woman I delivered had no pain and didn't scream at all. It was a very easy, uncomplicated delivery and I felt very chuffed indeed. I thought, this is it, a new life has arrived, a new entrant to the human race. It's a magical, emotionally charged event and it's one of the nicer aspects of medicine. You are involved in a very personal aspect of a woman's life.'

Another high point of the course was the month in casualty, where students saw the sharp end of emergency medicine and often had a chance to learn and practise practical procedures for the first time. St Mary's had a large, busy and well-organised accident and emergency department which not only provided formal teaching for students but also encouraged them to get involved in the treatment of patients. Jane Morris explained why it was so popular. 'It's really exciting and for the first time you feel useful. In casualty students are left to do things on their own and you realise that if you weren't doing the work somebody else would have to – and that makes you feel really worthwhile.'

During one of her night shifts in casualty, when all the other staff were busy, Dong Chiu was asked to stitch up a schizophrenic patient who had slashed himself in three places on his arm. Dong had practised the technique on tissue paper, but this was her first attempt at suturing skin. She began work at one o'clock in the morning and completed her twenty-fifth stitch two hours later. Dong was an accomplished dressmaker, but she said that sewing skin was nothing like working with material. 'Skin is very resilient. It was like sewing canvas with a needle meant for silk and the needle was curved, which made it very difficult to push through.' The work had been a challenge, but Dong found it satisfying to tackle the job alone in the middle of the night and complete it single handed.

Some of the other challenges facing students were less easily met and lingered in the mind for many weeks. Sarah Holdsworth had been a year in clinical medicine before she had to cope with her first death. She and another St Mary's student, Andy Taylor, had gone to a district hospital outside London for two weeks in residence with a firm of paediatricians. These periods of residence outside London were greatly appreciated by students since they were normally welcomed and valued by the firms they visited and given proper work to do. Paediatrics was particularly popular because children, oblivious to medical hierarchies, treated students as doctors. Sarah and Andy liked the hospital and the specialty and became very involved in the work of the children's ward.

One evening a five-year-old girl was brought into the ward after being knocked over by a car. She was put into the intensive care cubicle on the children's ward, linked up to a ventilator to keep her breathing and attached to various monitors. Sarah knew she was seriously ill but did not appreciate quite how seriously. The following day she and Andy took part in the routine ward round which eventually reached the little girl's room and everyone was standing round her bed discussing the case when one of the alarms went off.

'They realised her blood pressure was very low and started to check other things,' said Sarah. 'But everyone was very calm and matter of fact. Immediately afterwards the ECG alarm went off and I wondered what was happening. Then people just began to dismantle the monitors and remove the ventilator. I turned to Andy and whispered, "I think maybe this person has stopped being alive," and he said, "Yes." But no one else said anything, it was just completely routine. Eventually I said, "Is she dead?" and they said she was. And then the consultant went to speak to the parents who were in a room along the corridor, and suddenly there was this terrible wailing as they heard the news.

'Then someone said to me, "Come on, let's get on with the ward round," and they all went off to see the next patient. But I just couldn't go. My eyes filled with tears and I went off and sat on my own for a while to try to get myself under control. I kept thinking how she was at the age when children are so lovely, and of how much joy she must have brought to her parents' lives and how much they were going to miss her. I was terribly shocked by the experience. I'd been thinking that paediatrics was such fun, but I realised that bits of it aren't fun at all. I would have liked to have been able to just go away and cry, but you have to carry on – you can't run off in hysterics.'

Jane Morris commented on the lack of any counselling for students bruised by such experiences. 'You see terrible things and there is no one to talk to about them within the hospital. I'm lucky in that I've got people outside who I can speak to, but I've seen things that have really hit me hard.' In 1990 a confidential counselling service was set up for everyone working at St Mary's, including medical students, who wanted to discuss such problems, but few students seemed to be aware of its existence. Sarah Holdsworth phoned her parents every week and told them all she had seen and done. They felt she relied on them a great deal. 'Medical students need a lot more moral support than someone like our son who did engineering,' commented her father. 'There are lots of ups and downs that have to be addressed, and if your parents are not there backing you up, it could be quite lonely.'

Death featured surprisingly little in the curriculum. There were a couple of lectures in the pre-clinical course, a seminar organised by the department of general practice and an afternoon session during a week devoted to oncology – the specialty which covered all types of cancer. This session was held at the Pembridge Unit, an NHS hospice which had strong links with St Mary's, and it gave students a rare opportunity to discuss their experiences of death and to talk to terminally ill patients. Dr Anne Naysmith, the unit's director, said that students' exposure to death was very variable and, because of the way clinical teaching was organised, it was easy for them to avoid dying patients if they wished. When deaths did occur on the wards, they were generally treated in a matter of fact way and there was very little exploration of students' feelings. 'It is a very big gap in the education of most young doctors,' commented Dr Naysmith. 'You cannot teach students about death and dying in a single afternoon.'

A group of twelve fourth-year students who attended one of the sessions at the Pembridge Unit met Bernard, a man in his late forties who was dying of cancer and had only a few more months to live. It was a glorious spring day and sunlight and birdsong poured though the open windows of a seminar room as Bernard spoke about his illness in a quiet, unemotional voice. He described how he had attempted suicide after being told, bluntly when he was alone in an out-patients clinic, that his cancer had spread and no further treatment was possible. He also described recent episodes of total paralysis in which he had suffered agonising pain but was unable to move a muscle: the experiences had frightened him terribly and he was now scared to go to sleep in case it happened again and he died. (In fact he died peacefully a few weeks after he talked to the students.)

In a discussion after Bernard had returned to the ward, several students confessed that they worried a great deal about death, caring for terminally ill patients and breaking bad news, and felt that more time should be spent addressing these issues during the clinical course. All were conscious that they would have to look after dying patients when they qualified the following year, and they felt themselves unprepared. Several wanted to spend more time with terminally ill people in order to learn how to talk to them and many requested role-playing sessions with actors which would enable them to practise answering difficult questions or breaking bad news. 'Telling people that they are going to die is one of the very important things that we will have to do as doctors, and yet we hardly get any help with it,' said one student at the end of the session.

The quality of teaching varied enormously between departments and from firm to firm within the same specialty. Some departments were seriously committed to teaching and had devised a challenging progamme of lectures and seminars which filled students with enthusiasm for the subjects. Others seemed to regard students as an encumbrance. Good bedside teaching depended on the commitment of consultants and registrars. The system was something of a lottery: every few months lists were issued informing students which firms they had been allocated and, as Nick Hollings explained, everyone waited to see whether or not they had struck lucky. 'When the list goes up, it's a case of looking to see which consultant you have got and your heart either sinks or lifts. You either know you'll get a good deal or think: "I'll end up learning nothing."'

The Dean recognised the problem. 'There are some firms which fail to get students properly involved,' he conceded. 'But the good firms do expect students to be around and regularly clerk and present patients. However, an enormous amount is left to the enterprise and initiative of the students themselves and there is a limit to how much you can actually push them to get involved.'

The lack of uniformity in clinical teaching worried some consultants and moves were afoot to reform the curriculum at St Mary's. Mrs Margaret Ghilchik, a consultant surgeon at St Charles's Hospital, who taught students all year round, was a keen advocate of reform. 'The old apprenticeship system is out of date. There are too many students and too few patients in the London teaching hospitals for it to work any longer. I believe that, just as the ward round is becoming obsolete (it is horrible and degrading, for both the patients and the students), the time has come when the firm could also go.'

She wanted to see a more sophisticated approach, harnessing modern technology in order to make the best use of doctors' and students' time. 'All students should be given log books when they start the clinical course, containing a printed account of everything that's in the curriculum. They should be taught in blocks, when groups of surgeons and physicians come together to provide concentrated tuition on a particular subject, for example eyes or ENT, which are vitally important areas, but ones in which the consultants are too busy to manage apprenticeship-style teaching properly. There would be relevant patients, lectures, handouts, films and video link-ups to operations while they were in progress. We need to make our teaching fit for the 1990s: all that is required is someone to organise it – and that is what the professors are paid for.'

Mrs Ghilchik was one of only eleven female consultant surgeons in the country. A formidable woman in her fifties with a sweet but shrewd expression, she was famous in medical circles not only for having managed to breach the male bastion of surgery, but also for the superhuman feat of having given birth to four children without interrupting her work as a consultant. They were all born during her annual leave: on every occasion she continued operating until the day she went into labour, then announced that she was beginning her holiday, and was back at work exactly six weeks later. In the days before part-time consultant posts were even dreamed of, it was the only way to maintain a career in surgery.

For female students, Mrs Ghilchik was an inspiring figure – living proof that medicine and motherhood could mix. But they lamented the absence of more role models: there were only thirty-eight female consultants at St Mary's and St Charles's Hospitals out of a total of 170, and the women were concentrated in clinical jobs in the community or academic posts in the medical school. Half the students at St Mary's were now women, and when they entered medical school they were every bit as ambitious as their male peers, but as they progressed through the clinical course and learned more about the medical career structure, many began to worry about their futures as doctors. A glance at the employment statistics for hospital medicine revealed that women were still a disadvantaged minority. In 1988, when our students were beginning clinical medicine, only thirteen and a half per cent of consultants in England and Wales were women and in competitive, high status specialties their numbers were negligible. General and orthopaedic surgery boasted more than 1700 consultants, but fewer than one per cent were female; of the 1300 consultant general physicians, only five and a half per cent were women.

The Department of Health was committed to rectifying this imbalance, but the career structure of hospital doctors militated against the advancement of women, as Mrs Ghilchik pointed out. 'The registrar and senior registrar years coincide with women's reproductive years and the hours are simply dreadful: those who decide to have children at that stage have a terrible time.' Mrs Ghilchik was convinced that prejudice and resistance to reform of the hospital training structure accounted for many of the problems faced by women. Many female doctors complained of job discrimination and old prejudices undoubtedly persisted in some quarters. 'Some consultants seem to assume that women are of a lower calibre and will automatically go into general practice,' said Jane Morris. Halfway through her clinical course, Sarah Holdsworth commented, 'Medicine is sexist and so is Mary's. A lot of the older consultants trained at a time when there were very few female students and some of them believe that women shouldn't be in medicine. I can partly understand their point of view. They don't see why all that money should be spent training women who are then going to leave and have children. But women doctors have a lot to give.'

Although the Dean had not himself seen sexism at work, he recognised the problem. 'There are certainly members of staff who have been accustomed to living medically in a largely male society and whose attitudes reflect that. It is a different world for them now. I warmly welcome equality of opportunity in medicine. Women make absolutely first-class doctors, but our society puts them at a disadvantage by expecting that they will not only give birth to children but also take responsibility for raising them.'

Jane still hoped to forge a career in hospital medicine, but confessed that she was now keenly aware that her 'biological clock' was ticking away, she would have to think hard about how to fit in marriage and children: compromises would be inevitable. Sarah, like Jane, had grown up in a traditional family, with a mother whose full-time work was bringing up children, and she already felt torn between wanting to provide the same environment for any children she might have and the desire for a stimulating career. 'I know that it will be a time of conflict,' she said. 'I think it will be very frustrating. At the end of the day I will either do neither well enough or I'll do one well and leave the other one out altogether.'

For Ese Oshevire the problems were compounded because she was black. She believed she would face additional obstacles after she qualified because of her colour. 'There are racist people in every walk of life and medicine is no exception,' said Ese. 'I know that some consultants say to their staff, "If there are foreign names, just disregard the applications," so I will undoubtedly be discriminated against by some people because of my surname.' She had already experienced discrimination at St Mary's. 'I have been picked on at the medical school by a consultant and it came as a shock to me because it's the only real instance when I felt that someone really didn't like me just because of my colour. At first I thought it was just me, but then I talked to some of the other black students and realised that he has got something against black people. But it's very difficult to prove, and I knew I would come up against him in finals. I want to pass finals, so I said nothing. Whilst you are at medical school, there is very little you can do.' Ese's comments came as a shock to the Dean: racism, he said, was totally foreign to the spirit of the school. 'If I had known, I should have taken it very seriously and tried to do something about it.'

One source of stress among medical students was experienced by all, irrespective of sex, colour or class. During their first months of clinical medicine the students had to learn to ask probing personal questions and to conduct internal examinations.

David Copping outlined the problem. 'Having to do internal examinations, asking women about their periods and examining girls your own age when you are only twenty are huge hurdles of embarrassment. It is nerve-racking at the time and I think students could be better supported, but once you have got though it you start to feel more confident.' Gynaecology presented particular challenges, as Ese discovered. She enjoyed the specialty, but found talking to patients difficult. 'They want to speak to someone who knows what they are talking about and when I go up to them they look at me as if to say, "Oh no, I've got to tell all my problems to that little squirt." I feel on edge, because they are personal problems and I wouldn't want to talk to a medical student about them.' Ese found it difficult to break the ice and became embarrassed herself because the patients were clearly embarrassed. There were routine questions about sexual problems which had to be asked, but were feared by students and always left until last. 'You stutter and there's a big pause before you come out with something like "Do you have pain on intercourse?" Students received formal teaching on vaginal examinations and were given an opportunity to practise on women who were undergoing surgery and had received a general anaesthetic (the patients concerned had all given their consent), but Ese disliked performing the procedure. 'The patients are usually young women who haven't had children and aren't used to someone poking their fingers inside them.' She would have preferred to learn the technique thoroughly on life-size models.

Venereology, the specialty that handled sexually transmitted diseases (STD), was equally demanding. The department had a whole building to itself. The Jefferiss Wing, completed in 1989, was a testament to the importance of the Praed Street Clinic, said to be the biggest in Europe, which saw 70 000 STD patients a year. It also acknowledged the major role played by St Mary's in AIDS research. Students spent two and a half days per week there for a month, sitting in on the STD clinics and the Wharfside Clinic where HIV positive patients were seen. They also visited the hospital's two HIV and AIDS wards, where many met sufferers for the first time and learned how they managed their illness and coped with daily life.

The first visit to the Praed Street STD clinic was, by common consent, interesting but embarrassing. The clinic was so busy that scores of patients could be seen queuing in Praed Street before the doors opened in the mornings. It served a wide cross-section of people, from middle-class professionals in suits who dropped in on their way to work to prostitutes who worked in Paddington. Some of the stories they heard in the clinics shocked the students: Jane Morris recalled her amazement when a middle-aged man who had been married for over twenty years was asked how recently he had had a sexual partner other than his wife. He considered for a moment, then replied, 'Oh, it's been absolutely ages – it must be at least ten days ago.' Jane was also shaken by the number of young women she had seen who had been diagnosed as HIV positive.

In the clinics students were, as usual, expected to take histories from patients – but in venereology that meant a no-holds-barred sexual history including sexual orientation, favoured practices, frequency of intercourse and number of partners. Some simply could not bring themselves to ask the questions at first. Once the ice was broken, they had to learn to be completely non-judgmental, making no comment – either verbally or through their body language – as the patients talked. Male medical students were often asked to leave by female patients, so the women tended to get more clinical experience in the specialty. Sarah Holdsworth said she found the experience 'sociologically fascinating, but terribly embarrassing'. She recalled that when the senior registrar asked her to take a man's history on her first morning she was seized with terror. 'Well, actually I'd prefer not to,' she replied, 'because I can't tell who is gay and who's not and I might say the wrong thing.'

As the clinical course continued, the gap between our students and the patients they saw in clinics and on the wards widened. They began to develop a more professional manner, still friendly but also reserved, which enabled them to distance themselves from the suffering they saw around them. It was not uncommon to hear them talking about 'the gallstone in bed four' or 'the massive hernia in bed seven'. But a personal brush with serious illness could demolish those fragile defences. After two years of working on the wards, David Copping felt confident of his ability to cope with patients – until his mother was admitted to hospital. A healthy woman of fifty-one, she suddenly developed severe chest pain and an X-ray of the blood vessels around her heart revealed that one of her coronary arteries was almost entirely blocked. She was admitted to Harefield Hospital for an emergency heart bypass operation and David spent a lot of time at her bedside.

'This is the first time that anyone who is close to me has been in a life-threatening situation and it has taught me so much,' he said. 'It is upsetting to be on the other side, and see her as a patient with all the tubes coming out of her. It has made me realise that every patient is somebody's mother, somebody's spouse, and it will change the way I behave towards relatives.' He had watched his mother act out the role of the good patient in front of the doctors who were treating her. She had pretended to be fine and told them that she understood everything when she was actually nervous and worried about being cut open. 'Patients put up this front and doctors often tend to accept it because they are very busy and want to get on to the next patient. My mother's operation has given me an insight into this state of affairs and from now on I shall try to find ways of dispensing with the "busy doctor" manner in order to probe patients to find out what they are really feeling. 'You need to cut off from patients to some extent to survive, but you have to make sure that you don't cut off completely.'

Treading that path between empathy and professional objectivity was still difficult sometimes. There were parts of their medical training which took students into uncharted territory where it was difficult to formulate an appropriate ethical or emotional response. For example, there were some complicated and demanding procedures that could save life in an emergency, but which were too dangerous for students to perform on live patients. The only way for them to learn was to practise on people who had just died. No one doubted the educational value of these sessions, but many students found them deeply disturbing. David Copping had to put a central line (a very fine bore tube which is inserted into a vein near the collar bone in order to deliver fluids and drugs direct to the heart) into a man whose heart had just stopped beating. 'It can be a life-saving procedure, so we have to practise it, but it is an awful thing to have to do,' said David. 'I just concentrated on what I was doing and didn't think about the person – but I won't forget it for a long time.'

For many students, the most gruelling episode of the entire clinical course was an afternoon teaching session on termination of pregnancy. It took place every week at the Samaritan Hospital, ten minutes' walk away from St Mary's, and students were invited in pairs to watch abortions being performed in one of the gynaecology operating theatres. The surgeon was Mr David Paintin, reader in gynaecology at St Mary's and a lifelong campaigner for liberal abortion, who had helped draft the 1967 Abortion Act. The session was not compulsory, but most students chose to attend. Towards the end of their first year on the wards Sarah Holdsworth and Nick Hollings made their way to the operating theatre: neither was looking forward to the afternoon. Eighty-seven per cent of abortions in Britain were performed before the twelfth week of pregnancy, but the Samaritan specialised in the remaining thirteen per cent: they were going to watch late abortions.

Nick and Sarah changed into theatre gowns and went into theatre where they stood on either side of Mr Paintin as he worked. He explained the surgical techniques involved, and sought to place the procedure in its social and ethical context. Typical patients were young teenagers who had concealed their pregnancies, he said, and some were the victims of incest. They arrived at the hospital with pregnancies of eighteen weeks and beyond, pregnancies which could not be terminated in the usual way because the foetus was too large. There were two options for gynaecologists: surgery or induction of labour. At the Samaritan they dealt with late terminations surgically: this involved giving the woman a general anaesthetic, dilating her cervix, then destroying the foetus inside her uterus and removing it in fragments through the cervix as it was too large to be removed in one piece. Mr Paintin regarded the alternative method – the induction of uterine contractions by drugs – as barbaric: the mother would have to undergo labour and deliver a dead foetus, a process that would be deeply distressing for her, those attending her and other patients on the ward. The procedure they were watching was, in contrast, distressing only to those in the operating theatre.

Nick and Sarah saw several terminations during the afternoon. The most disturbing case involved a girl who was twenty-one weeks pregnant. Both turned away from the operating table from time to time, exchanging glances and screwing up their eyes in distress as Mr Paintin removed the foetus bit by bit. He told them that abortion was very common in Britain: more than 150 000 pregnancies were terminated every year and at least one in four women between the ages of fifteen and forty-five had had an abortion. 'It is a very common problem in general practice and gynaecology – and that means that doctors have got to think their positions out in advance. Both doctors and patients share an unease about the morality of abortion which persists even among those of us who have been doing it for twenty-five years.' Mr Paintin told them that his understanding of the social and emotional problems of the patients who came to him with unwanted pregnancies provided the moral framework for his work. 'I find that knowing the situation of the woman and the distress she feels makes it possible for me to do terminations without feeling uncomfortable. I believe I am doing a proper thing, helping her with a major problem in her life. It doesn't feel like an immoral act.'

Afterwards, in the surgeons' tea room, Mr Paintin discussed the ethics of abortion with Sarah and Nick and asked them how seeing the terminations had affected them. Nick said that the experience had been upsetting because he had been able to identify parts of the baby's body. 'You could see limbs, fingers and ribs. I'm not particularly squeamish and I don't have any strong moral feelings about this procedure, but actually seeing identifiable parts of the body made me think: this is a prospective human life here which has now been terminated, and perhaps one should think about it again a bit more carefully. From a moral and humane standpoint, it's the most moving thing I've seen.' Both students emerged from the session convinced that gynaecologists should do such work in order to prevent the return of back-street abortions, but for the moment, neither felt they would be able to participate. Sarah was visibly shaken by the experience. 'I have a problem with abortion and I find it very disturbing. It is a very necessary thing, but in my mind it's still the destruction of a life. I don't think I would ever be able to rid my mind of the feeling that I was killing something. When you see a baby being born, the hands are really cute because they are very small and grasping. And here you see a little hand coming out and it's not moving, which is really distressing, because it was never given a chance.'

Despite the fact that she was deeply upset, Sarah had no regrets about attending the session. 'I think it's important to see it. As doctors, we are not here to sit in judgement on women. If I become a GP and patients come to me for help I will refer them for abortion. When you see things like this it expands your personality and builds your character. It makes you a more sympathetic person and you become a little bit wiser than you were before. It is the most shocking thing I have seen at medical school and I shan't ever forget it.'

John Shephard, who watched the session with two other students, said afterwards, 'The consultant said it would be unpleasant and he was quite right. It was the most stressful time of our careers. My group started fooling around and we had to be told to be quiet. We don't normally behave like that – it was a response to the stress. I don't know how the consultant does it, week after week.'

These stresses and strains of clinical medicine were, for the most part, suffered in silence. There was only one teaching session during the entire clinical course which was designed specifically to examine students' feelings about medical school and their prospective careers. It took place in the department of general practice: students spent two weeks with GPs in practices all over the country, then two weeks having seminars, discussions and video-consultations where they acted as GPs and actors played their patients. On the final afternoon they attended a session entitled Self-Care in which one of the course tutors invited them to take a hard look at themselves.

The seminar started slowly: students were unused to voicing fears or revealing weaknesses, but gradually they began to talk about what it was like to be a clinical student. They felt they did not have a proper role and that too often they roamed the wards in search of something useful to do. Ward teaching was seldom timetabled and sometimes seemed to happen at the whim of the consultant. Several students said they had felt humiliated by senior doctors during ward rounds and many felt that they had been exposed to traumatic events during the clinical course with little warning and no support. Encounters with seriously ill or dying people often left them feeling drained and helpless. Other pressures on them came from society at large. Trainee doctors were expected to be mature, responsible and selfless: pillars of society. They were also expected to like all their patients, even when they were dirty, smelly, rude and annoying.

The tutor, Dr Derek Chase, produced statistics which showed that the health and happiness of doctors could be seriously compromised by the stresses of the job. Male doctors were three times more likely than other male professionals to become alcoholic, get divorced, or commit suicide. Divorce and suicide were seven times more likely among women doctors. 'We are a pretty sick bunch in medicine. The pressures will always be there and the statistics are a worry. Of course it always happens to somebody else, but *someone* has to be the statistic. Life is going to be tough, and in order to deal with the quagmire you are in you have to look after yourselves.'

Everyone had different coping mechanisms. Ese Oshevire had managed to keep up her athletics throughout medical school and was glad to have an interest which took her right away from medicine. She was an outstanding athlete who specialised in the heptathlon, which consisted of seven events and took up two days during competitions. Ese had to train most days in order to maintain her standard. Her short-term goal was to become Britain's number one heptathlete; long-term, she hoped to compete in the Olympics. Will Liddell escaped the pressures of medicine by climbing mountains; Dong Chiu had many creative interests including drawing, sewing and photography. Mark George and Nick Hollings played golf and went drinking with friends. They had shared a flat a few minutes' walk from St Mary's with two other students throughout the course and both said that having a home outside the medical school contributed substantially to their sanity. Fey was forcibly removed from the stresses of medical school by the competing demands of home and family and seemed to achieve a balanced existence as a result.

Jane Morris and Sarah Holdsworth were heavily involved in the dramatic life of St Mary's, performing in plays and musicals throughout their time at medical school. In 1989, they directed the St Mary's soiree, which was both an escape from and a celebration of the myriad stresses of medicine. Held on the last Saturday of term before Christmas, the soiree was a kind of institutionalised anarchy – an annual opportunity for the least powerful members of a formidably hierarchical organisation to flex their muscles and dance and sing out of line, insulting their elders, betters and patrons. It had a reputation for being bawdy, offensive, immature ... and most of the students seem to love every minute of it.

The soiree indicated how far our students had travelled since their initiation during Freshers' Week. Then, they were raw recruits, given a glimpse of the future through the jocular Norfolk Lecture, but barely understanding the jokes. Now, they were insiders who had broken the taboos surrounding illness, naked-ness, sex and death and it was their turn to make the jokes. Sarah and Jane introduced the evening's entertainment. They had per-suaded an unusually large number of consultants to participate, including the Dean, who teamed up with Dr Oscar Craig to contribute a song and dance routine. 'The place is heaving – it's electric,' Sarah said. 'When it's your turn, everyone is looking at you, at your humour, your personality. It gives me a massive buzz, much more than any other kind of acting I've done.'

Sarah was the author of 'The Dead Patient' sketch in which Will Liddell appeared as a brusque, sarcastic consultant and Sarah and a friend played two hapless medical students. Between the students and their teacher stood a hospital trolley on which repined what appeared to be a corpse covered by a sheet – though only a single motionless arm was visible. What followed borrowed heavily from the famous Monty Python dead parrot sketch.

Will: 'This is an ex-patient. She has gone to the great out-patients in the sky.'

Sarah: 'No, Sir, she's just not very talkative.'

And so it went on, the jokes in progressively worse taste and progressively better received, until the evening was over and Sarah and Jane collapsed in a euphoric heap backstage and reflected on the secrets of their success. 'It's like a club,' said Sarah. 'You only get the jokes because you're part of the medical profession, people outside don't understand them. It gives you a very nice feeling. The humour is notoriously about medical situations we have all been in – so everyone can relate to it. Everyone remembers the consultant making them feel a fool and can relate to the sketches. The crudity and jokes about parts of the body come from an overfamiliarity with human anatomy: we're dealing all day long with things that are taboo for normal people to talk about and we discuss them without batting an eyelid. And that breeds jokes.

'Take the dead patient sketch. Someone came up to me afterwards and said, "That happened to me on a ward round." People will probably think that's terrible and upsetting, but in actual fact you do laugh in that situation – not on the ward, but to yourself. You think: this is ridiculous, here we are standing round the bed ... and the patient's dead. It's so typical of a teaching hospital ward round, where the consultant doesn't really notice what is going on with the patient and the students don't either, because they are so busy trying to find out the information and haven't looked at the patient properly because they are so nervous. You're not laughing at the person because he's dead, but at the funny situation we are all in.'

6

FOREIGN LANDS

'The elective period of study is one of the highlights of the undergraduate course. It provides an opportunity for you, usually during your fourth or fifth year at medical school, to spend part of your course (about eight weeks) to travel abroad or remain in this country in order to broaden your medical education.' BMA Medical Students Group booklet.

When Will Liddell banged his leg he thought nothing of it. It happened on a boat trip in the eastern part of Papua New Guinea as Will was halfway through his elective, those two happy months away from St Mary's to which he and every other medical student had been looking forward for years. Events like the soiree provided temporary relief from the rigours of clinical study, but the elective was a real break, a long break, probably the only one they would have for years. They could go wherever they liked in the world, provided their medicine would benefit. Most students chose to go abroad. In theory they hoped to see patients with rare illnesses and diseases in their most advanced forms. In practice many looked forward to an extended, exotic holiday.

It was summer 1989 and Will was having a tremendous time, travelling around the Pacific islands, taking part in health clinics. 'I'd usually go out with a nurse in a boat and we'd visit villages. One day we walked for two hours through a coconut plantation and a mangrove swamp to do a clinic. When we arrived, someone would blow a big conch shell and we would wait, usually under a mango tree in the middle of the village, for the mothers to come along with their under-fives. We'd weigh all the children, then examine and vaccinate them and give them vitamins. It was a new experience for me to be asked to make clinical decisions, especially in the absence of a qualified doctor, but I consoled myself with the thought that, though I might not do anyone any good, I was unlikely to cause harm. I really enjoyed that: it was the most gorgeous place, completely cut off from the Western world.' The cut on his leg was to lend an extra dimension to Will's elective. Although he dressed it carefully, it became infected, and a few days later, when he was out celebrating his birthday, it began to hurt very badly.

'It became very swollen and soon I couldn't walk on it. By the end of the evening, I was feeling very cold and realised I had a fever,' recalled Will. He spent a sleepless night poring over medical textbooks and wondering what was the matter. The following morning, a doctor from the local hospital was called to examine him and immediately admitted Will to hospital and put him on a drip. The diagnosis was septicaemia or blood poisoning, a potentially life-threatening illness, and Will was very seriously ill. 'Luckily they had the appropriate antibiotics and I got better in about a week,' said Will. 'But I was pretty ill and quite frightened, because my textbook listed all the complications of septicaemia, some of them fairly nasty.'

In retrospect, Will felt that this episode of ill health had been the most educational part of his elective. 'I was very well looked after, but from the point of view of my medical training it was almost the most useful thing that's ever happened to me. It's not an experience which I would ever like to go through again, but it does make you realise how frightening it is to be in hospital and just how rotten you can feel when you've got bacteria floating round your bloodstream.'

Peter Richards, the Dean, believed that the elective was a vital stage in the education of medical students. 'They learn how well off we are for medical care in the developed world and how peripheral many of our ideas about medicine are to the health of underdeveloped countries. And they come back even more resourceful, independent and mature.'

Students were asked to submit their proposals to the medical school, but few were turned down. They spent many evenings poring over maps and reading the elective reports of previous students before making their choices.

When Ese Oshevire began to plan her elective, she set herself some guidelines. 'I want to go somewhere sunny and hot, where I can see rare cases. Somewhere where I can do my athletics and where I won't be discriminated against. I have experienced discrimination in the past and I don't want to go somewhere where I would feel like an outsider.' Because of her family connections, Ese had spent a lot of time in Africa, and she did not want to go there again, but she had always wanted to visit Jamaica – and her long-term boyfriend Simon Stacey wanted to go too.

Ese's elective was fairly typical in that it began at a central hospital, with the student shadowing a handful of doctors, and continued in a more rural, less medically sophisticated, part of the world. The hospital in Kingston, Jamaica's capital, was a low, modern, circular building set against a backdrop of bare hills. Ese and Simon reached it via an eye-opening ride from the airport which took them past Kingston Bay with its stunning scenery, past mango sellers, sunbathers, a thousand ghetto blasters and walls festooned with political graffiti.

At first glance, Kingston General seemed very similar to any British hospital. The worried faces in the waiting room, the patients being wheeled about on trolleys, the announcements over the Tannoy. Ese started her elective in the paediatrics unit, where she was briefed by a consultant, Dr Morrais. What did Ese hope to gain by her time in Jamaica? It was two years since she had done paediatrics, Ese replied, and she would like to brush up on the basics and to see how the Jamaican approach differed from that at St Mary's. Ah, but the medical school at Kingston is based on the British system, replied Dr Morrais, almost reprovingly. Ese brushed a few flies off her face and carried on listening. She was impressed by the standard of care at the hospital. 'It's not second best here. It's absolutely top notch.'

After a tour of the wards, Ese sat in on an out-patients clinic, having quickly refreshed her memory of paediatrics by glancing at the *Oxford Handbook of Clinical Specialities*. She immediately noticed that all the children were immaculately dressed as if going to a party. In fact, in Jamaica everyone dressed up before visiting hospital and Ese found it impossible to guess their background.

A little later at the swimming pool, over a glass of orange juice, Ese and Simon were filled in by Professor Edwin Besterman, a resident Englishman and retired cardiologist from St Mary's, about medicine in Jamaica. It quickly became clear that there were substantial points of difference between St Mary's, Paddington, and Kingston General. Because of the lack of a national health service in Jamaica, Professor Besterman explained, patients reported to the hospital in a much more advanced state of disease than in Britain. They came to the hospital because it was cheaper than going to see a family doctor. The hospital used the American names for the various grades of doctor: housemen were called interns, registrars were residents. And there were other nuances of language. ...

'Country people have a certain dialect and you must speak slowly. A foot goes all the way up the leg. A belly goes up to the chest. You want a man to take his vest off, he won't know what you're talking about. You have to call it a marina. If you ask a patient how far he can walk he won't answer you in yards, he'll use chains. A chain is 22 yards. And they won't be short of breath, they'll blow.

'Here you'll see patients in gross heart failure who've never been near a doctor before. Ankles swollen, enormous livers, totally emaciated. You don't see this at home. Here you see it in the clinic every Friday. Half our medical beds were knocked out by Hurricane Gilbert and we've still got a quarter of them not back in action. So we send patients home who would horrify you in England.'

Why had he chosen to retire to Jamaica? 'Because my training was in advanced heart disease and I think I can help more people here than I can in the UK. I can do it with a stethoscope and I don't need hi-tech.' It sounded like a permanent elective; Professor Besterman was obviously happy in his work.

Ese found the Jamaican medical students very friendly and easy-going. 'They're just like us, really. Trying to skive off at any given moment.' After a week she felt pleased with her decision to come to Jamaica – 'just a little disappointed that the hospital's not nearer the beach.' Simon was also enjoying himself. He had discovered some Welsh rugby players and a decent supply of beer.

A few weeks later Ese left Kingston and moved up country to the small town of St Ann's Bay. There three remarkable doctors worked long hours in difficult conditions to keep a 120-bed community hospital running. The hospital was a collection of one-storey whitewashed buildings with verandahs. This was hospital medicine in the raw.

The maternity ward had been built as a TB ward thirty years earlier. It now handled 2600 deliveries a year, Ese was told, and had beds all down the middle of the ward as well as four in the corridor. There was a rapid turnover and women went home twelve hours after delivery. There were generally more patients than beds and women in early labour normally shared a bed. There were no foetal monitors to record the condition of the babies during labour. When several woman approached delivery simultaneously, Dr Hall, the English obstetrician who ran the unit single-handed, had to run from bed to bed to attend them. He explained that patients held their own notes – and rarely lost them – because doctors were not always available.

One sad, but, for Ese, particularly interesting case was that of an old lady with breast cancer. She had gone to hospital with a lump and a biopsy had shown it to be malignant. The hospital sent a telegram asking her to return, but the woman would not come; she said the lump was not hurting. By the time she did return, seventeen months later, the lump had ulcerated on to the surface of the skin and had to be cut out. Drugs and radiotherapy were given to prevent the spread, but the prognosis was poor. The woman would live about two years. Ese assisted at the operation, 'holding the odd scissor here, and snipping the odd thing there'. Such an advanced cancer was rare in Britain.

Half the population of Jamaica was under twenty-one and consequently the children's unit at St Ann's Bay was particularly hard-pressed. One ward was full of emaciated children suffering from malnutrition. Dr Betton, the paediatrician, asked Ese to guess the age of one tiny, wasted boy with swollen ankles. 'Four or five?' she hazarded. 'Fourteen,' replied the doctor, explaining how sustained malnutrition had left the child permanently physically and mentally handicapped.

Most of the work at St Ann's was what Ese called 'grass roots, do-or-die medicine. The type of medicine that everyone likes to do: hands on.' The doctors at the hospital seemed to have great job satisfaction: they were doing the kind of work she had dreamed of when she decided to enter medicine.

Back in Kingston, at the casualty ward of the Public Hospital, Ese and Simon found themselves dealing at first hand with the urban, discontented face of Jamaica. The hospital served the whole city, including its roughest quarter, Trench Town. There were stab wounds, head injuries from people throwing stones, gunshot wounds, motoring injuries, as well as a lot of referrals from rural areas. Within hours Ese was trying hard to remember how to suture as she stitched up a boy with a head wound. He was followed by a man in a similar condition who had been fighting over a screwdriver and was 'cut by a cutlass'. The ward was full of screams and groans; a woman cried for water; a twenty-one-year-old woman had been shot in the back by her baby's father because she hit him on the head. 'I've never seen a gunshot wound before,' said Ese, surprised at how small the hole was. 'It depends on the distance,' explained Dr Taylor, the young casualty resident. She told the students that they would learn a lot at the hospital. 'You'll get a lot of experience and learn to manage without high technology.'

The casualty ward changed Ese's views about Jamaica. 'Overall I think it's a really nice country, scenic, beautiful, friendly people. Up until today I was really getting to like it. I felt I could live here. But there's always a dark side to life and it's a real eye-opener to see how easily people just get angry and violent over just simple things. This hospital's near to Trench Town, a ghetto area. People tell me that some of them compare scars, but I think it's just a release of frustration, anger, everything.'

'I think as a doctor you can become cynical. I don't feel like that yet. I can see both sides of the coin and I still feel very sympathetic, very emotional really, although I don't show it. I

suppose the move will come when I am in a position of responsibility.'

One thing Ese particularly enjoyed during her elective was
being a black person in a black country. 'I just feel part of the
furniture here, and I don't get stared at: it's really nice being
anonymous.' Simon's experience of Jamaica had been very
different: he had felt like an outsider, said Ese. 'You could say it's
like me at home but I've lived with it all my life. He's had all the
prejudices at once, you know, people calling him "whitey", even
if they were just joking.'

The elective had given Ese time to think about her career and
crystallise her ambitions. What she really wanted to be was a GP
in an inner city. Her experiences in Jamaica had made her realise
that people could change things. 'All you have to do is make
yourself part of the system that runs the problem, and you can
start to alter things. The best place to be to change the inner cities
is right in the middle.'

For their elective, Jane Morris and Sarah Holdsworth had chosen
a really exotic location: the Solomon Islands. Twelve thousand
miles from Britain, it was one of the most expensive elective
destinations. The trip cost them £3500 each (including the price
of a round-the-world air ticket), most of it paid by their parents.
They had chosen the Solomons because they had read that they
were beautiful and unspoilt. They were also conveniently situated
for visits to Australia, New Zealand and Tahiti. Sarah and Jane
had looked forward to the trip for months, but their first
impressions on arrival in the capital, Honiara, were negative.

No one in the hospital seemed to know who they were or what
to do with them, and they were kept waiting before being directed
to their living quarters. To their horror, they discovered that their
accommodation was already inhabited – by rats, cockroaches and
several thousand mosquitoes. 'It was only our lack of understanding of the Solomon telephone system that prevented us
bringing our flight forward by seven weeks!' commented Jane.

Four days later they had fallen in love with the place. They
were taking part in a survey to find out the prevalence of hepatitis
B in Guadalcanal Province, which involved a four-day journey

by plane, tractor and boat to reach some of the most remote villages in the islands. They often had to jump out of the canoes some distance from the beach, holding medical supplies above their heads, and, because it is taboo in the Solomon Islands for women to show anything above calf level, they had to wade through the deep water while fully dressed. The presence of two white women was obviously a rare occurrence in many of the villages, and consequently Jane and Sarah attracted crowds of giggling children wherever they went. But the hordes rapidly disappeared when they brought out their syringes. Sarah took blood samples while Jane performed the hepatitis vaccinations and Nelson, their Solomon Island nurse, reassured the villagers to 'have no fia, small nila – lack moskito, im strap yellow eyes.' ('Have no fear, this small needle is like a mosquito that stops hepatitis.')

After three weeks in Honiara, the girls flew to Gizo in the western province where they had arranged to work at the local hospital for four weeks. 'Gizo was the best part of the elective,' said Sarah afterwards. 'It was the nearest place to paradise you could ever find.'

The hospital, while being of a very high standard in third world terms, came as something of a shock to them. The beds, less than half a metre apart, were covered with stained old mattresses and pillows that looked fit only to be burnt. The wards were fly-infested, hot and smelly. They worked every morning from eight until lunchtime. The morning's work began with the ward round, a slow and laboured progression around the beds. 'We've seen some good pathology as people really don't present with their affliction until it's serious – and consequently too late,' said Sarah. 'This is partly because the Western Province is a collection of widely dispersed islands, so it's a major operation to transport themselves by motor canoe to Gizo.

'We're becoming adept at diagnosing malaria and TB simply because *everyone* has malaria and TB, and often both. There are some shocking spinal injuries caused by falling out of trees, cutting trees down and falling head first through the cargo hold on a ship, to mention a few. One young man has completely transected his spinal cord and is now paraplegic, incontinent, with bed sores and severe wasting of his legs. The worst part is that there's nothing that can be done for him, as there are no rehabilitation centres, not even one physiotherapist in Gizo. The best we can do is to ensure he opens his bowels, passes urine and remains free from fever while his father just sits quietly with sad eyes, watching him.'

Hepatitis was one of the greatest problems in the Solomons and one night they admitted a young man with acute hepatic failure probably due to the disease. Sarah had never seen anyone so ill. 'The whites of his eyes were yellow and his liver and spleen were huge – all textbook stuff. He needed a liver transplant, but what could we do? We can't even do the basic liver function tests in Gizo. By the next morning he'd slipped into a hepatic coma and his whole family assembled to begin the mourning process. Eerie cries could be heard throughout the whole hospital, with his mother throwing herself prostrate across his body. On went the awful wailing. I don't think I'll ever forget it. Then they took him home to die. There's none of your "inform the coroner, ring the mortuary" stuff here. The family simply takes the body back home to rest in peace.'

Out-patient clinics were held every day and operated rather like casualty in Britain. Patients were often referred from their own village clinics and the nurses dealt with seventy per cent of them, leaving only the serious cases for Jane and Sarah. In order to take histories and treat patients, they had to learn the rudiments of 'pijin inglish'. Functional enquiries were limited to basics such as pain, eating, drinking, vomiting ('You thro out?'), diarrhoea ('Garum bellerun?'), bowels opening ('You sits it good?'), and passing urine ('Mimi gud?'). One of the most commonly used sentences seemed to be 'Me no savie' (I don't know). Some of the translations of medical terms were picturesque in their literalness: for example, if Jane or Sarah wanted to perform a vaginal exam-ination, they would ask the patient: 'Me lukim baskit blong pikinini?'

'You can never hope to understand the patients' replies to questions,' commented Sarah. 'So you become adept at inter-preting nods, grunts and eyebrow movements and end up exam-ining just about everyone. Once you have learned the limited list of obsolete drugs available off by heart, you're all set – we hand out prescriptions left, right and centre.'

After a hectic morning of examinations, translations and prescriptions, Sarah and Jane would return home for lunch and spend the afternoon diving on the coral reef. Both had taken a course in scuba diving and they were addicted. Sarah described the sensation. 'As you glide down through the depths there's a magical feeling of weightlessness and for forty minutes there's nothing to concern yourself with except schools of exotic fish which swim right up to your face. When you look up, you can see the silhouettes of all the fan-shaped corals and literally thousands of fish above you.'

When their stay in the Solomons came to an end, Sarah and Jane took a holiday. Sarah met up with four other St Mary's students who had gone to south-east Asia and the Pacific for their electives. Meanwhile Jane's boyfriend, Tony Gilbert, flew to Australia to join her for a fortnight. She had met Tony, a solicitor, eight months earlier and had introduced him to her parents just before she left for the Solomons.

During the last week of the holiday Jane and Sarah travelled to the Cook Islands and Tahiti together. While they were there, Jane made an announcement. Sarah recalled the scene. 'We were lying in bed one night talking before falling asleep when, suddenly, Jane sat up in bed. She said: "Sarah, there's something I've just got to tell you – I can't keep it secret any more. Tony's asked me to marry him and I've said yes."'

Jane was surprised to find herself contemplating marriage at the age of only twenty-three, but two months apart from Tony had strengthened her conviction that it was the right thing to do. She thought marriage would inevitably change her and alter her priorities. 'I feel less driven now than I did at eighteen. When I started at medical school, I was ambitious without realising the cost of achieving my ambitions. Now I have seen what you have to go through to succeed in hospital medicine and I'm not sure I am willing to do it. I don't want to risk my marriage.'

Some students eschewed exotic locations and primitive medicine and chose instead to attend centres of excellence in Britain. Fey Probst was one of them. She needed to stay in London to care for her four children and in any case she could not afford to travel far. She spent her elective at the Clinical Research Centre at Northwick Park Hospital in Harrow in the department of psychiatry. Most of her time was spent collecting data for a research study designed to identify families in which at least two brothers or sisters had schizophrenia. She chose the place and the project partly for career reasons and partly for convenience.

John Shephard also chose his elective with an eye to the future. He had travelled widely as a naval officer, like Fey he was studying on a tight budget, and he thought it would be unfair to leave his wife behind, so he opted to go to two of Britain's most famous hospitals: the Brompton, in west London, where the Egyptian surgeon Magdi Yacoub was doing his pioneering heart transplant work, and Great Ormond Street, the world-famous children's hospital. His decision was motivated by ambition: John wanted to make a career in hospital medicine and electives at the two hospitals would enhance his c.v.

John had been lucky to be accepted at the Brompton and was instantly impressed by Professor Yacoub. At once autocratic and charismatic, he carried out his ward rounds accompanied at all times by his secretary, a medical Boswell who not only held his stethoscope but also took down every word he said in shorthand. John was also astonished by the surgeon's energy. It was not uncommon for him to operate in three countries in as many days, and the Brompton list was often done in the evening after he had jetted in from the United States, France or Egypt.

John's month at the Brompton was everything he could have wished. He received a lot of one-to-one teaching from Magdi Yacoub and learnt, for example, to strip veins from the leg for use in a heart by-pass. The highlight of his time there was a trip by private plane to Dublin to collect a heart for a transplant. 'The transplant organs had to come from within four hours' travelling distance of the hospital in order to keep them in good condition. We had a nine-month-old child coming from Liverpool, who had to wait until an organ became available. I was in the National Heart and Lung Institute Library when I was grabbed to go with the senior registrar from Harefield to Dublin for an organ. The heart was stored in a cool box packed with ice and we had four hours to get it into the child. It was a bit of a race against time, but we made it with fifteen minutes to spare. The operation was a success and when I last heard the boy was doing very well.'

Medical students were a bit of a rarity at Great Ormond Street. Most visitors were either postgraduates or foreign doctors but after writing 'a considerable number of very begging letters', John had managed to arrange an attachment to the department of haematology, which cared for children with blood disorders, including leukaemia, and the department of oncology, which dealt with all types of cancer.

John was allowed to devise his own timetable and he decided to start with out-patients clinics and graduate to the ward. Almost all patients at the clinics, he found, had been in-patients at the hospital. Most were now having shared care: they normally visited their local district hospitals, but returned to Great Ormond Street regularly for a battery of tests to check that their illnesses were completely under control. These visits were tense times for the patients and their parents. They had to be prepared for news of a relapse or the discovery that complications had set in. Many also had to have chemotherapy injections to treat their cancers, which they dreaded.

In 1989, when John was at Great Ormond Street, the Wishing Well building programme was under way, following the extremely successful appeal (£52 million was raised). The hospital was covered in scaffolding and plastic and conditions were more cramped than ever as whole departments moved into temporary accommodation so that building could begin.

John met several parents whose children were terminally ill. Their stories were often harrowing and he discovered that it was impossible to attempt the history-taking routine he had learned at St Mary's. He learnt more by simply sitting back and listening. 'You can go a long way through medical training,' he explained, 'without meeting the full emotional impact of what disease means to other people. Only paediatricians come face to face with what it really means to have a fatally ill child. How do you cope when you meet that kind of tragedy every day?'

His elective had confirmed his interest in hospital medicine and he felt he had benefited enormously. 'Technically I've learnt more about leukaemias and haematology. I've also learnt a lot about myself and about children. Paediatrics is the most interesting thing I've met in medicine. It's given me a new insight into sickness. You realise that children are central to people's lives and you are the only person who can provide a cure, which is a big responsibility.'

By now John was veering towards a career in paediatric surgery, a remarkable ambition in a man who was already thirty-two. He would not qualify for another year, and would then have to serve about ten years in the specialty before he stood a chance of becoming a consultant. He would be at least forty-three before he achieved his ambition, and the competition along the way would be fierce: there were only sixty-five consultant posts in the specialty.

John had by now been been married for twelve years. His wife Debbie had been a vital prop throughout his time at medical school. She continued to live in their house in Plymouth during the week, working as an estate agent in order to support their household. John tried to return home most weekends, but during the clinical years that was not always possible: sometimes he had to be on take on a Saturday night or attend a weekend ward round. He frequently paid tribute to her and said that without her he would never have stayed the course. But he acknowledged that his medical training had put a strain on their relationship. 'Medical school hasn't been the doddle we thought. The emotional cost has been high. Debbie has watched me change quite a lot and sometimes she worries that I may go off her. She has invested a tremendous amount in all this, putting off having a family and going out to work. I worry that we'll grow apart to the point that we cannot relate to one another, and medicine would not be worth that. I would hate to lose her. Luckily we have the sort of marriage that can survive these kinds of things – so I think we'll be safe.'

Mark George, like John Shephard, wanted to have a career in hospital medicine, but he had time on his side. He chose an elective destination that offered a 'brilliant holiday' as well as teaching that would help prepare him for finals the following summer. Mark went to the University Hospital in Cape Town with another St Mary's student. They opted to spend their first month in the department of obstetrics and their second with the neurologists. Obstetrics was one of the four subjects examined in finals and Mark knew he needed to revise it thoroughly; in Cape Town the teaching was excellent and he felt on top of the subject by the end of his stay. After their time in South Africa the two students went on safari in Kenya for a month.

Our remaining three students, David Copping, Nick Hollings and Dong Chiu, all went to Sarawak in east Malaysia – one of the most popular elective destinations. Nick went with two friends from St Mary's. He chose Sarawak because it was off the usual tourist track. 'It seems sensible to really make an effort to go somewhere outside the everyday destinations. You don't want to stay in Europe; I didn't particularly want to go to the States; I've been to Africa; so the Far East seemed like a sensible option.'

He had begun in the capital Kuching, at Sarawak General, a large hospital with more than 700 beds where he did three weeks paediatrics and two weeks medicine. The staff all spoke English and were very friendly, and, as Ese had discovered in Jamaica, the standard of the consultants was just the same as that at St Mary's. The city of Kuching had been friendly, but there was the usual Third World contrast of international hotels situated just a few minutes away from shops that looked like hovels, selling huge bunches of bananas for about four pence, as Nick put it.

The highlight of Nick's elective was a trip up the Baram River with one of the VHTs, or Village Health Teams, consisting of paramedics but no doctors, which took medical care to the tribal peoples. The VHT travelled up river through the forest in ever-smaller boats as the water got progressively more shallow and spent the nights sleeping in the longhouses – literally long wooden houses – where the villagers lived. Each evening a member of the team gave a lecture on a common disease like malaria or dengue fever and the next morning they held an out-patient clinic.

Nick enjoyed life in the longhouses. 'It's very hot and noisy, you drink a lot, never go to bed and watch kung-fu movies at all hours, but it's very hospitable. Any chance of a party and they take it. Sleeping takes second place.' In many ways it resembled Nick's life at St Mary's.

The journey up the river was uneventful, past a succession of settlements, each with a prominently-situated church. The rain forest was being devastated by logging companies and the river trip brought Nick face to face with extreme contrasts. 'It's a real mixture of undisturbed, beautiful thousand-year-old jungle and man's relentless progress. Looking across the river now, I can see a large swath of forest completely wrecked. There are piles of logs on the river, the water is filthy and every ten minutes or so a logging boat charges past. In a place like this they are in the dark ages and in the twentieth century at the same time.'

The first village they reached was new, wood-built and dominated by the jungle, its looming canopy providing a spectacular backdrop for the misty mornings and huge yellow sunsets. The longhouse was the focal point of the village. The all-important headman lived there, as did many of the families, and the clinic was held there too, in public. Nick was impressed with the dedication of the VHT and the one-to-one nature of the health care. Henry Penrigan was the team's senior medical assistant, a young, lively local paramedic who treated the morning clinics almost as theatre, but clearly knew what he was doing. The patients waited on a bench before being summoned to a red chair in front of the doctor.

There was a woman with an infected thumb, another with a thyroid problem, a third with chest pain. The fourth patient, an old Kayan woman, wore a wonderfully colourful flat hat and ornamental weights that stretched her earlobes in a string of skin down below her shoulder blades. Her forearms were heavily tattooed and she wore a pink T-shirt with the legend, 'Ha! My dinner!' Medically, however, she was a relatively uninteresting case of high blood pressure. It wasn't until the fifth patient came in that Nick found himself taking a blood sample for a case of what could have been malaria.

They continued along the muddy river to another village, Long Keseh, a small distance up the Baram by the flat-bottomed, pencil-shaped boat, about 1.5m by 12m, that had become a second home. The journey was enlivened when the team encountered rapids and had to get out and push the boat. Basic sanitation means a lot here, and that, as Nick discovered, was all down to the local headman. In Long Nakon there had been running water, television, videos; in Long Keseh there were none of those things. The reason was that until 1985 there had been only one community, in Long Keseh, but in that year half the people had followed a new and evidently more dynamic headman down the river.

Many of the patients were suffering from work-related diseases, but as Nick put it, 'It's very difficult to find out what's going on here because the system is totally different. In England patients sit or lie down, you know what you're doing, and you go through symptoms in a specific order. Here there's no time to do that, they're sitting there, there's no bed, and you have to think immediately "What is this likely to be?" and then go straight to whatever you think is wrong and ask the relevant questions. Again that's difficult because you've got to go through an interpreter so you can't pick up the nuances of the conversation.'

Instant diagnosis was a challenge, but not one that tempted Nick. 'I wouldn't want to carry on medicine in this way. You can easily miss things. It's impossible to examine an abdomen properly when someone's sitting up.' He nevertheless had great admiration for the health teams, most of them committed Christians, who visited the longhouses once a month – and a growing under-standing of their problems. Many of the local people, for example, had cataracts which were probably diabetes-related. Diabetes could be picked up early with a blood sugar test, but to get the villagers to monitor their own blood sugar would require more frequent visits. Instead, the health teams had set themselves simple targets, concentrating on preventative medicine. There were lec-tures on dengue fever, malaria, cholera, and lessons on healthy cooking, the importance of boiled water and birth control.

Nick's trip up the Baram and back took three and a half days. He slept uncomfortably on concrete floors, ate more chicken and rice than was good for him, and took part in at least one traditional dance in which he was forced to don a feathered cap and tunic and carry a shield and sword. Was it worth it? What had it taught him? 'Not to take anything for granted. And as regards medicine, to be a bit more incisive, not dawdle around.' He had also acquired a kind of intuition for what might be wrong with a patient. 'When you're taught as a medical student how to clerk people, I think very little emphasis is given to using your senses and picking information up. You're taught to go through a check list, and you're so busy remembering which question comes next you're not actually thinking.' Now Nick was beginning to pick up signals using his eyes and ears, even his sense of smell.

The elective had also enabled him to put his career into focus. He had seen a lot of palliative treatment, and for him that did not seem enough. He was veering away from general practice and towards hospital medicine. As he put it, 'It's more fun in a way to deal with people who are acutely ill, knowing "OK, I've got to do this right. If I don't it's curtains. But if I get it right, I've saved a life." '

David Copping also went to Malaysia, spending most of his time in general practices in villages around Kuching helping in community health programmes. He quickly realised that inspecting the sanitation of a village could be a greater contribution to the health of its inhabitants than any quantity of medication: clean toilets and fresh water were fundamental in the fight against disease. David said he had seen advanced leprosy for the first time, but overall had learned more about public health policies than medicine.

He travelled to Malaysia with his wife Karen, having joined the small band of married students six months earlier, at the beginning of his fifth year. He had met Karen, a physiotherapist who trained at St Mary's, the previous year and they originally planned to get married after finals. Then David decided to do a one-year clinical BSc degree which would have postponed the wedding for two and a half years. 'We don't believe in living together, so we decided to get married the following summer,' said David. 'Marriage has a very poor image at medical school and lots of people said I was making a big mistake. But I don't see it as settling down, simply as making a monogamous commitment to someone I love.'

Dong Chiu flew to Sarawak alone, but received a huge welcome at the airport. Her elective was very different from those of the other students: she had been born and brought up in Kuching and was returning home for the first time for three years. Some 300 000 people live in Kuching and about half of them are Chinese. Dong's family were among them. Her parents lived in a comfortable villa on the outskirts of the city. They had raised four children and all of them now lived overseas: one daughter was a pharmacist in Australia, another was a fashion student in London and their son had followed in Mr Chiu's footsteps, he was a civil engineer in Indonesia. Dong's parents had prepared a feast for her and soon after her arrival her family were tucking in, with chopsticks. Dong, as if to emphasise her individuality, used a spoon, and informed her family that she hardly ever ate meat now. They were alarmed and told her it was unhealthy to go without meat: as a trainee doctor, she should know better.

Dong's parents had great faith in her commitment to medicine. She had announced that she wanted to be a doctor at the age of five, they said, and her mother had bought her bulls' eyes to practise dissection, which Dong had loved. Her father thought she would eventually work in hospital medicine. 'She does things quickly and wants to see more and she is curious. She would be stifled in a small place.'

Shortly afterwards, Dong, like Nick Hollings, found herself in Sarawak General Hospital, trying to understand her first patient in the radiology clinic. He was speaking in Bahasa, though it could equally have been English, Chinese, one of the many variants of Malay, or a tribal language. Like many patients he had a nasopharangeal cancer, which was common in the Far East and resulted in the growth of a tumour around the nose and throat. To get to the hospital the man had had to sell two of his fighting cocks, but, because he was very poor, the hospital would not charge him for treatment. He was doing well: radiotherapy had reduced the size of his tumour.

The next patient was less fortunate. He had a huge swelling on his neck, produced by the same type of cancer, but it was in a very advanced state. He was a fisherman from a remote village who had lived with the cancer for months before seeking medical help. Even now, he did not always turn up for his treatment because he had six children to support. Now bone scans showed that the cancer was spreading throughout his body and a cure was impossible. The doctors in Kuching faced a dilemma: should they continue with his treatment a little longer, or send him home to die while he was still mobile?

The third patient was an old woman with a swollen jaw. For fifty years she had been chewing betel nuts and now she too had nasopharangeal cancer. Each nut was about the size of a hazelnut and she used one a day, broken into small pieces, mixed with a white lime liquid and rolled up in a green betel leaf. It was the lime that had caused the cancer. With treatment she had a fifty per cent chance of survival over five years. After the clinic Dong slipped a little betel into her handbag. 'I'm going to have a try,' she confided with a smile. 'It can't hurt me, not just one little try.'

Her next adventure was with the flying doctor service which provided medical care for all the villages that could not be reached by the Village Health Teams. The doctors tried to visit each village once a month, and the service's three helicopters were stretched to their limit. As she flew six hundred metres over the Borneo jungle – 'like watching a Vietnam movie' – Dong had a graphic view of the effect of logging on the landscape. Everywhere there were crooked strips of white in the green of the trees, roads made by the logging companies; and where the lakes were still blue, the rivers, starved of oxygen, ran brown. Dong's reaction was mixed, 'On the one hand, it's a great shame, a bad idea. On the other hand, the Malaysian economy depends on the logging. I think the way they've done it is not correct. They've devastated areas, leaving them scarred with soil erosion.'

Today the helicopter team were paying a visit to the Penan people. She had learnt about them in books at school. They were nomads, hunters, who made clearings in the forest which they cultivated for a while before moving on, always in a circle. At least, that was how it used to be. Now the Penan worked for the logging companies and stayed put.

The health team set up an out-patient clinic in the longhouse at Long Itam. Dong had just begun to examine the patients with a young female doctor when the helicopter was summoned to an emergency. The pilot took off alone, but returned almost immediately. With him in the cockpit were a young couple and their little daughter. Dong and Dr Singh ran across the grass to the helicopter, but it needed only a cursory examination to establish that the child was already dead, a victim, like so many others, of diarrhoea. For this little girl, modern medicine had arrived too late. If she had been given fluids and essential salts, she would have lived. Dong explained later, 'I might have tried to resuscitate the child, but we didn't know how long she'd been dead, and if we'd brought her round she might have been brain damaged. It would have been very difficult for her parents to cope with her in a setting like this. Back in England, a crash team would undoubtedly have resuscitated her, and there would have been support available if she was handicapped as a result. But in the jungle, it is the survival of the fittest. It is difficult to accept, but you have to face reality.'

Back in Kuching, Dong reflected on her elective. Would she be tempted to come back to practise medicine in Sarawak? 'There is a lot of work to be done here and lots of preventive medicine, but the lack of facilities would be very frustrating. It would be nice to come back here with a mobile operating theatre for the people who cannot get to hospitals, but that requires a lot of money.' If she did return, she thought it would be important as a doctor to throw one's weight behind demands for more money for medicine and better living conditions for the people.

In many ways Dong Chiu had been as much of a foreigner as the other St Mary's students when she visited rural Sarawak. 'Malaysia is a lot more interesting than I had thought. I spent most of my life stuck in Kuching and never went to the jungle. During my elective I have got to know my own country. It has opened my eyes.'

7

THE FINAL HURDLE

After three months in paradise, London and the monochrome familiarity of a British winter appeared particularly unattractive to students returning from their electives. In halls of residence and rented flats, they swapped photographs, regaled one another with tales of life in the bush and tried not to think about what lay ahead. They knew that their return to St Mary's marked a turning point: the carefree days of sports, soirees and parties were coming to an end, to be replaced by months of slog. The immediate prospect was specialties and senior firms – the final part of the syllabus. Six months to a year away hovered the ghastly spectre of final examinations. In between, students had to find out about and apply for their first jobs. There was a daunting amount of work to be done.

The period following the elective was recognised as one of the low points in the medical school course. Everyone found it hard to settle back into the routine. Sarah Holdsworth, who had celebrated her twenty-third birthday on the Barrier Reef, now sat at her desk in a rented house in Shepherd's Bush on a dull, damp December morning and confessed to feeling very miserable. 'On the graph of enthusiasm, I am fairly near the bottom at the moment. I feel more unsettled than I have for a long time.' After an absence abroad, the British medical scene looked bleak. Friends recently qualified reported long hours and low pay; and recent changes in the organisation of the NHS had produced shock waves so strong that they had even reached medical students, normally impervious to such events. 'The political situation has made us all down in the dumps. We hear all the consultants saying, "Well I'm jolly glad I'm retiring soon," because it looks as though they are not going to be their own bosses any more. And I think to myself: that's great, I'm just starting.'

There was nonetheless some relief that the course was in its final stages: five or six years is a long time to spend in one place. Even Jane Morris, who had been heavily involved in the artistic and social life of the medical school, felt it. 'Mary's can be a bit claustrophobic. There are only a hundred people in a year, which boils down to twenty who become close friends; and now we're the oldest and there's no one new to get to know,' she said. 'I'm glad it's coming to an end.'

Part of the frustration lay in coming back to the same institution and the same role. Many students had tasted real responsibility on elective. Even those who had stayed in Britain reported that they had been treated as useful members of the team and had felt more central to patient care. Now they all found themselves back in wards, out-patient clinics and theatres as observers: sometimes taught, sometimes ignored, frequently bored. This was the last opportunity for students to acquire the theoretical knowledge and practical skills required to qualify as doctors and the remainder of the course was designed to help students revise. Two weeks were spent with a firm in obstetrics and gynaecology – though many students felt this was a woefully short revision period for a subject that loomed so large in finals and which they had last studied two years earlier. There was a third and final attachment to medical and surgical firms, with students spending six weeks in each and, sandwiched between them, a fortnight of anaesthetics.

Anaesthetics was regarded as a postgraduate specialty and students needed only a rudimentary knowledge of the subject for finals. Most, however, looked forward to their short stint in the specialty. Each student was assigned to a consultant and given one-to-one teaching – several said this was the first time they had enjoyed such a luxury in five years. They were shown how to perform the magical feats of anaesthesia: putting patients to sleep, eliminating their pain, relaxing their muscles and taking over their breathing; then restoring breath and consciousness perfectly on cue, just as the surgeons tied their last stitches. They learned the rudiments of obstetric anaesthesia and about pain clinics and the leading role played by anaesthetists in the intensive care unit. They liked the fact that they were allowed to do intricate practical tasks such as inserting a breathing tube into the patient's trachea (windpipe) and placing a breathing mask over the face and maintaining respiration by rhythmically squeezing an oxygen-filled bag. Anaesthetics also provided a golden opportunity to learn for the first time, or in some cases revise, a whole range of basic intravenous procedures: inserting catheters, putting up drips and administering drugs, which they would have to perform countless times as qualified doctors.

After Christmas in their final year students began to apply for the house officer posts, the crucial first rungs in their career ladders. Few had ever applied for a professional job and they were unfamiliar with the ritual, but the majority had attended a lecture on the subject at St Mary's which offered tips to the uninitiated. The speaker, Dr Andrew Vallance-Owen from the British Medical Association, explained that technically the under-graduate course did not end with the final examinations. When they graduated, the General Medical Council would provisionally register them for one year while they worked in recognised pre-registration house posts. During this first year, graduates were expected to undergo further training and assessment. Then, pro-vided their consultants considered that they had reached the required standard, they would become fully registered with the GMC and entitled to practise as doctors.

The normal pattern was to do six months each of general medicine and general surgery, though other combinations were possible. Dr Vallance-Owen suggested that those who wanted to make a career in hospital medicine (and especially in surgery) should try to find a job in a teaching hospital. Six months in a district general hospital would provide far more practical experi-ence, but the references, support and contacts available from a professorial unit were vital to a hospital career. He told the students to ignore competitive gossip. 'There is always someone in every year who has allegedly had the professorial house job sewn up since the pre-clinical years. What often happens is that everyone thinks the job has already gone, so no one else applies.'

A well-presented curriculum vitae was vital. So were good references, which played an invisible but critical role in the careers of doctors. 'A bum reference is a disaster, so do not ask people, "Will you give me a reference?" they may do so and it may be terrible. Ask, "Will you support me with a reference?" which will force them to say whether they will actively support you – few people will lie if you ask them like that. It's not just a matter of a written reference; you need referees who will lobby for you and ring up on your behalf.'

St Mary's, like all medical schools, had a pool of eighty recognised pre-registration house jobs for its graduates. Some were at St Mary's, St Charles's and Central Middlesex, others were scattered throughout England in district hospitals as far afield as Dover, Rugby and Hereford, where consultants had links with St Mary's. Six months before their final exams, students were asked to select eight of the jobs in the Mary's scheme in order of preference. Their choices were then computer matched with consultants' preferences and two days after the final results were announced, the list of house officers would be posted in the medical school.

The more ambitious students quickly realised that house jobs were vitally important if they were to get their careers off to a good start. They were about to enter the cut-throat world of medical patronage – a world in which who they knew would be every bit as important as what they knew.

Mark George and Nick Hollings hoped to forge careers in hospital medicine. Mark wanted to do cardiothoracic surgery, an extremely competitive specialty, and he therefore applied for two top surgical house jobs at St Mary's, in the hope that he would have a good and relevant reference from a prestige firm before applying for a surgical SHO job in a year's time. Nick's first choice was a popular and high-status job on the professorial medical firm at St Mary's. He too appreciated the value of a good reference, though his career path was less clear: he knew he did not want to do general practice or psychiatry, but general medicine and anaesthetics both appealed.

David Copping's priorities were very different. His wife Karen was working as a physiotherapist at the Brompton Hospital and they wanted to stay in their flat in Kilburn, so all his eight choices were in west London. He was worried nevertheless that the computer might ignore his selection and banish him to a hospital in the shires. David was the only one of our ten students who was absolutely certain about his long-term plans. 'Before I came to Mary's, I always pictured myself as a GP and that hasn't changed. I like being my own boss and I think general practice is more amenable to family life. I'd like to be part of the community, rather than behind a white coat, and involved with families and continuity of care. It's a very hard thing to be a very good GP, but that's my ideal. In ten years' time I'd like to be in a group practice of five or six doctors in the south of England, looking after patients from all kinds of backgrounds. I'd like the practice to be linked to a church.'

For the first time in five years, students were in open competition for the best house jobs and the atmosphere in the medical school was palpably different. Friendly familiarity was replaced by secretiveness: a widespread tactic was to elicit the job choices of other students in order to apply for good, but undersubscribed posts. There was an abundance of rumour and gossip. It was widely held that popular, gregarious students, who had played a lot of sport (thereby getting to know consultants socially) and involved themselves enthusiastically in the life of the medical school, would have the pick of the jobs at St Mary's. Some said that, in order to maximise the impact of an application, it should be handed to the consultant in person. This belief condemned several students to an exhausting chase which sometimes lasted days.

Ese, who had now decided against general practice and was keen to have a career in sports medicine, had applied for a job on a firm of orthopaedic surgeons at St Charles's and had talked to both consultants on the firm. Her c.v. included an impressive list of achievements in athletics: she was named as London University's Sportswoman of the Year two weeks before she sat finals, was now ranked thirteenth in Britain in the heptathlon and hoped to continue her demanding training programme while doing her house jobs. In her interview at St Charles's she was asked the inevitable question, 'Which comes first, medicine or sport?' and worried that firms might discriminate against her because she would need to take time off to attend competitions. At a subsequent interview for her fourth choice job at Hillingdon Hospital, another candidate told her she had already fixed up her second house job, in Ascot. Ese, puzzled, asked her how. 'Oh, the consultant who runs the firm is a friend of my family,' came the confident reply. Ese smiled knowingly and looked away. 'It's all right for some,' she murmured.

Some students did not apply for jobs through the St Mary's scheme, preferring to find their own posts at hospitals further afield. Will fixed up a job in Bath because he knew and liked the area and wanted to work in a district general hospital in order to get a broad level of experience. He thought he would be less of a dogsbody than contemporaries who had opted for teaching hospital jobs. John Shephard had arranged a job at Derriford Hospital, ten minutes away from his home in Plymouth. John already knew where his heart lay in medicine, but was uncertain whether he could fulfil his ambitions because of his age. 'I like acute medicine which is black and white, where you have to make decisions, and I would dearly love to be a surgeon. Being in theatre is almost recreational for me, but it is very competitive and at thirty-three I don't know whether I'm too old to enter the rat race.'

Once they had despatched their house job applications, there was little to divert students from the business of qualifying. The final examinations were a horrendous prospect. Some medical schools evaluated students by a mixture of exams and continuous assessment, others spread the exams over several years. But at traditional medical schools like St Mary's three years' work was assessed by the time-honoured method in eleven theoretical and practical exams spread over a three-week period. Students were examined in four subjects during finals: medicine, surgery, clinical pharmacology and therapeutics (drug treatments for illnesses and their effects), and obstetrics and gynaecology. There was a three-hour written exam for all four subjects consisting of hundreds of multiple choice questions and essays, but most of the marks rested on the clinical exams and the vivas.

Clinicals tested the candidates' ability to examine patients and work out what was wrong with them. Students were given one long case and several short cases. For the long case, they were introduced to a patient and left for forty-five or fifty minutes to take a history, conduct an examination and come up with a differential diagnosis. When the time was up, the students had fifteen minutes to present the patient to two examiners in a separate room, rather in the manner of a ward round presentation, and were then quizzed about the findings and the management of the patient. This was followed by three or four short cases: the examiners took the candidates to see several patients and asked them to point out the physical signs of their illnesses and arrive at a diagnosis. There were three clinical exams – in obstetrics and gynaecology, medicine, and surgery–and any disease or condition that was in the textbooks might turn up in the examination room.

Vivas were held in all subjects – and lasted twenty minutes. The range of possible questions was limitless. They could be specific, requiring students to identify anatomical specimens or pieces of equipment, or open-ended, posing clinical problems and asking the candidate to outline a plan of action: a man comes into casualty complaining of chest pain and you are called to see him, how do you approach the problem? Students would be expected to discuss history taking, examination, investigations, possible diagnoses and avenues of treatment.

The volume of work required to cover the examination syllabus was so huge that it displaced almost every other activity. Most students began revising in January or February, four or five months before finals, building up to an intensive effort from Easter onwards. Nick Hollings was typical: he worked for three hours every evening, after returning from the hospital, and for six or seven hours a day at weekends. He had given up all exercise and when he was not working felt consumed with guilt. Most of his work took place at a desk in his bedroom, where scores of books and files spilled over the floor. Nick estimated there were a thousand sides of handwritten notes and several books to be revised. 'There's so much to do that, no matter how hard you work, you've never done enough. When you get to finals, for the first time no one tells you what you need to know. It's like being in a chronic anxiety state and it's very hard to keep your motivation going. There is so much to learn that cramming is useless: you have to try to go through everything at least twice using a mixture of long-term and short-term memory. You cannot hope to learn everything by heart so you just have to hope that you'll start to recognise patterns. For example, in the clinical exams, you think hard about the implications of the patient's age, sex and social class because that narrows the possibilities considerably.'

Mark George, Nick's flatmate, agreed that he had cut back his active social life substantially in order to put in several hours' revision every day. (He came back from retirement briefly but gloriously in March to score one of the winning goals in the final of the London Hospitals Hockey Cup.) Mark's parents lived in Hertfordshire, less than an hour's drive from Paddington, and most weekends he went back to the house where he had grown up. While his mother did his week's washing, Mark might play a game of golf or croquet with his father, before heading upstairs to the study to put in a few hours at his books. He was worried by the amount he had to do. 'Basically, I'm trying to catch up on three years of clinical medicine,' he grinned. 'And that means I've had to make a set of notes and settle down to learning them. This is the final hurdle, and it would be a shame not to get past it.'

The students matured in a sudden and surprising way during the last six months of the course. They changed from laid-back undergraduates to focused, highly motivated professional trainees, hungry for information: one began to believe they would soon be doctors. Nick Hollings put it well. 'There has been an incredibly steep learning curve for the past four or five months, where we've gone from knowing practically nothing to hopefully knowing enough to get through finals.' If so much progress could be made in so short a time, was the course perhaps too long? Nick thought so. 'I think you could knock a year off the clinical course and still pass. We could have easily done it in two years.'

In addition to the final firms, the medical school organised a series of revision lectures which took place one day a week for the final three months. But this part of the course was not regarded as useful by the students, as Sarah Holdsworth explained. 'We are supposed to have lectures all day, but at least fifty per cent of them haven't happened because the lecturers just haven't turned up. It's a complete waste of our time.' Some medical schools provided a full-time revision course in the months before finals and many said they would have liked one at St Mary's. 'I think they should organise tutorials for us with senior doctors teaching small groups for all the different subjects,' said Sarah. 'That way, everyone would have an equal chance.'

In the absence of such a formal revision course, final year students were forced to fend for themselves and most arranged teaching sessions in their own time. Typically, groups of three or four students would approach registrars and senior registrars five or six months before finals and ask them to teach them on a regular basis – usually once a week for two or three hours. This practice had been followed for as long as anyone could remember and students fought for certain key figures who were known to offer excellent teaching and preparation for finals. No money was involved: the teachers did it out of interest, altruism and a desire to ensure that at least some of the final year students were competent when they started on the wards as their house officers in a few months' time.

Jane Morris and Sarah Holdsworth were both in groups which had fixed up seven or eight hours of extra teaching per week and when they heard, through qualified friends, of interesting patients in other hospitals, they would drive miles to see them. They both deplored the competition and secrecy that surrounded private teaching. 'Certain people go out and grab as many teachers as they can and people who are a bit slow off the mark have no one,' commented Sarah. 'Competition is mounting and little cliques are forming round the hospital. It would be very easy to get psyched out by it all. I'm glad I don't live in a hall of residence – I don't have to put up with everyone talking about work all the time.'

John Shephard, who had arranged five hours of tutorials every week, agreed. 'The competitive element is very repulsive: lots of people play psychological games, running through lists of all the extra tutorials they are having to make everyone else feel they are missing out. But it's no use expecting to be spoon-fed – this teaches you to be self-reliant.'

Mark, Nick and two friends had arranged numerous extra-curricular teaching sessions with senior registrars in several specialties. They had approached their teachers in the December before finals and the sessions began in January. They travelled into central London for some teaching: to Great Ormond Street for paediatrics and to the National Hospital for Nervous Diseases for neurology. Dr Robert Logan, a research fellow in gastro-enterology and a sought-after teacher, saw the group for two hours every week to coach them in medicine, therapeutics and exam technique. He estimated that students needed to know eighty to ninety per cent of the syllabus to pass finals, and said that medicine, the biggest subject, was probably the hardest to revise. 'Clinical medicine has no set text. Surgery is easier in that half of it is operative technique, which no student is expected to know for finals, so they only have to concentrate on diagnosis and management. Medicine, in contrast, is a huge area, which it is quite impossible to cover completely. It's like an ever-receding horizon: when you think you've reached the end, there's more stretching into the distance.'

He encouraged students to change their approach to taking histories from patients for the three clinical exams. 'When they start on the wards it's very easy to regard history taking like filling out a long questionnaire,' he explained. 'Now they have to draw conclusions rapidly, as they question the patient, and I see my role as helping them to collect and prioritise information efficiently.' He taught the students to interpret signs and symptoms quickly and process the information they had gathered. 'At the beginning of the clinical course, they took hours to take details from the patient and work out what was happening, but in the exam they have forty-five minutes to take the history and fifteen minutes to present it. The skill lies in making a precis of the patient information and putting it in a logical order. It's like being a journalist: working out what the story is, verifying it, then telling it in the right sequence. Everything they say in the presentation has to be relevant and safe.'

Nick Hollings abandoned the checklist approach six months before finals and found he now arrived at a diagnosis much more quickly. 'It can be very satisfying: sometimes you can get the diagnosis after they've said only two words. It's a matter of cutting through the rubbish and going straight for the jugular.' His average history-taking time before establishing a firm diagnosis had been forty minutes before he started revising – now it was down to twenty. Consultants could often manage it in two minutes, he remarked ruefully.

The student's manner with patient and examiners was all-important because, although a basic level of knowledge was essential, the exams were designed to test whether or not the candidate would make a competent house officer. Most medicine would be learned after qualification: at this stage they were expected simply to have the basic tools for the job. Good communication with the patient was vital and students strove constantly to improve their style by practising presenting patients to senior doctors who then criticised the performance. Confidence was all-important: every candidate's nightmare was to become flustered over an error or omission, lose concentration and collapse under the gaze of the examiners. Much of the teaching in the final weeks was devoted to polishing presentation skills in order to make such a disaster less likely. Students were urged to look at the examiners, not the patient, when presenting. They were told to refrain from nervous ticks, to be concise and never to say 'presumably'.

Dr Logan was a seasoned observer of the examination scene, having taught final year students for five years. He described how 'finals atmosphere' permeated the medical school: all social life came to a halt and the students began to approach their work differently. For the past three years they had worked on their own, but now many were firmly established in groups in order to give one another moral and practical support. A common practice was the simultaneous 'gutting' of several textbooks: each student would take one of the standard works on a subject and summarise it in note form for the group, so that, in effect, each student had read several books.

All students felt nervous and uncertain as finals drew nearer, but Dr Logan tried to offer reassurance. 'I say to them, "If you feel worried, look at your year and think of five people who are worse than you: they are the ones who will fail. There are always one or two people who deserve to pass yet fail, and I see my job as making sure that you are not one of them." I tell them to get themselves into a group and to stop living alone and move back into hall. I have no sympathy with people who don't get themselves organised into groups for extra teaching: they have been at medical school for five or six years and it's up to them to organise themselves.'

Dong Chiu was one of the few students who spurned additional teaching because she regarded the whole business of clubbing together and competing for teachers as 'terribly cliquey'. But this meant that she had to work entirely on her own. 'It could help to work in a group: two or three heads are definitely better than one,' she said. 'But I feel a bit inhibited about going up to registrars or senior registrars on my own and bothering them.' She had started her revision in late March but, recalling the debacle of her first-year exams, feared she might have left it too late again. She managed anything from nought to six hours' work per day. Dong believed people failed finals because of lack of knowledge, and therefore concluded that theory was the most important thing to absorb. She revised by imagining a patient walking into a clinic with particular symptoms and worked out the differential diagnosis – revising a whole host of things in the process. She was scared of having to examine patients in front of people. 'I can do it in my room, but during an exam situation, the whole thing breaks down.'

The patients who featured in clinical exams were of two kinds. Some were ordinary in-patients who were clinically interesting and sufficiently well to endure a morning of interrogation and examination by terrified students. But there were never quite enough suitable patients on the wards, so the organisers turned instead to ex-patients who had been called upon on previous occasions. These were the so-called 'professional patients', veterans of medical exams who trotted out their histories succinctly and chronologically, often using the appropriate medical terms they had heard so often. It was said that, if they liked a candidate, they would divulge all the relevant information without any prompting. Indeed, in the previous year's finals a female patient had handed a student a tightly-folded paper containing full details of her history, diagnosis and treatment. Such patients were the stuff of dreams.

For 'ordinary' hospital patients, the run up to finals could be a nightmare. At a time when budget cuts were forcing wards to close, the number of in-patients was lower than normal. But almost one hundred students, whipped into a fever of clinical activity by peer-group competition, were desperate for people to practise on. It was by no means unusual for an interesting patient to receive visits from twelve students in one day, all anxious to question him exhaustively and conduct a full examination. Given that most hospital inhabitants are ill and tired, their level of compliance was heroic. But as the clinical exams drew closer more and more of them could be heard saying weakly, 'If you don't mind, I'd rather not, you're my fifth group of students today and I'm not feeling very well.'

The students with cars drove out to new pastures. Luton, Kingston, Watford: wherever there was a whisper of a ward full of varicose veins or a hospital doing hernias they followed the call like bird-spotters, hoping to glimpse common medical and surgical cases that were now rarely seen at St Mary's. Surgery was particularly badly hit: operating lists were frequently cancelled owing to the shortage of beds, and the London teaching hospitals no longer contained the cross-section of cases seen in an average district general hospital. Beds were filled by patients with rare and exotic conditions, and the bread and butter cases which came up in finals were thin on the ground.

The Dean was sanguine. 'There may be more clinical students in London than there are opportunities, but when we have a substantial part of north-west London at our feet, there is no shortage of patients. We have got to increase the academic contribution of outlying hospitals, where there are plenty of patients, and we need to extend the clinical skills teaching beyond the hospital setting. But every medical school in the country is in the same situation.'

Four weeks before the exams began, the final-year students laid aside their books and stethoscopes, donned dinner jackets and party dresses, and set off for an evening of unbridled enjoyment: the Final Year Dinner. The event, held at the medical school or in a nearby hotel, was organised by the Students Union, which also invited consultants who were popular with the students.

'This is the last thing we'll do as a group before our final exams,' said Will Liddell as he adjusted his bow tie in his Notting Hill flat, 'and I think everyone realises that it's the end: we're not going to be medical students for much longer. The dinner is a significant occasion – a bit outrageous and a bit nostalgic. People want to relax and let off some of the steam that they've been bottling up since they started revising for exams. There's also a major life event coming up: we're going to start work as qualified doctors soon.' The evening began with a champagne reception. Then came dinner, which was accompanied by speeches from students and consultants. Afterwards there was dancing and drinking until three or four in the morning.

The last three weeks of the course were not timetabled and most students went home to revise for part of the time. Will Liddell spent several days with two other students in a remote cottage in the Lake District, then went to his parents' farmhouse in Hampshire for the week before the exams. He worked in the conservatory where the only sounds to disturb his concentration were the bleating of lambs and cawing of rooks. It was late May, and the scent of elderflower filled the air. Will spent his mornings working and the afternoons fly fishing on the river that flowed through the farm. 'I think it is important to give your brain time to concentrate on other things,' he explained. 'I'm sure that subconsciously I am still processing the information, but there is only a certain amount I can do in a day. If the fish aren't rising I sometimes take a little pocket book of questions in obstetrics and gynaecology and quiz myself.'

Will was quietly confident that he had done enough to pass and was looking forward to working as a doctor. He was now fairly sure that he wanted to be a GP. Ploughing through notes and textbooks during finals revision had made him realise that he did not want to take any more major exams (which were obligatory for a career in hospital medicine). In addition, he had realised that working directly with patients was the aspect of medicine which most interested him. 'Looking back on the course as a whole, I'm less intrigued by the more mechanistic aspects of medicine than I am by the emotional and social aspects, and general practice is what brings those kind of things to the fore.'

Most of Fey's revision took place in the very different circumstances of her chaotic house in east London. She was surrounded by children: playing, fighting, squealing, making Lego models, doing homework. When she returned home from St Mary's at half-past four, Fey, now separated from her husband, had no time to relax. She had to cook supper, inquire about four separate schooldays, supervise homework, play and read, before dispatching her brood to bed. Catherine, the eldest, normally disappeared at ten o'clock and Fey did housework until midnight. Only then could she settle down to work, usually for two or three hours. She admitted that it was almost impossible to revise with the children around. 'I think they feel they have to compete with my work. It's as if they are saying: "Mummy, if you love me, put the books away."'

Catherine, now aged thirteen, described the domestic pressures facing her mother with detachment. 'She rarely manages to revise enough for exams because of us. The night before an exam she doesn't let us stay up at all, then once we have gone to bed, she works until about three in the morning, trying to make up for what she hasn't done through looking after us.' Fey seemed to cope with the competing demands on her time with admirable nonchalance. She had an unerring sense of the priorities in her life, tremendous stamina and the capacity to concentrate briefly but hard. She acknowledged failure as a possibility, but was convinced that, even if she came unstuck first time round, she would pass at the resits.

John Shephard was less relaxed. During the final weeks he looked pale, tired and nervous – and admitted he was terrified. 'I know that I'm good on the wards and can do the job, but I don't know whether I've taken on board the quantity of information that I need. Underneath this confident exterior, I'm just a common dog sailor and suddenly I feel I have no right to be here. I'm not an intellectual, but I'm surrounded by intellectuals and I wish I were cleverer. It's very hard competing against the youngsters, who seem to have this tremendous capacity to absorb information. I think I've done well to take on board the general concepts and they come out with the fine detail. It would be very embarrassing to fail.'

Finally the exams began. First came the written papers, and students gathered outside the examination hall as they had before first- and second-year exams, exchanging anguished smiles and desperately making conversation. They looked older and far more drawn and pale than they had in their pre-clinical years: a testament to months of voluntary imprisonment.

Clinicals and vivas, which followed a week later, were more demanding than the written papers since they required a polished, multi-faceted performance from candidates. It was not enough to cram facts and regurgitate them. Now they had to behave like competent, confident, well-prepared doctors. It was received wisdom that arrogance, rudeness to patients and scruffiness could result in failure. All the candidates were dressed as if applying for consultant jobs: men in suits and blazers, their trousers creased razor sharp and shoes gleaming, women in suits or sober-smart dresses. They had suddenly aged ten years. Their dress and deportment exuded knowledge and confidence. Unfortunately many of them looked as if they were about to be sick.

There was a degree of solemnity and ritual surrounding the clinicals and orals. The exams were held behind closed doors and the examiners hunted in pairs: their names were posted outside. Silence enveloped the anteroom where the exam organiser paced up and down, stopwatch in hand, bell at the ready, waiting to signal that time was up. Candidates waited there, two at a time, tying knots in their stethoscopes and whispering commiserations to one another. John Shephard, waiting for his surgery viva, confessed to a fellow candidate, 'I have never been so stressed, so consistently, for such a long time. I can't think of any other job that imposes this kind of stress just to get in at the bottom.'

Ese said the finals were much worse than any previous exams she had sat because they went on for so long. 'I've been worried for months. I can't sleep, I can't eat, I feel sick all the time.' She felt she had fallen down in her medicine clinical but insisted that basically, she knew how to do the job. 'Finals are like the driving test: you know that you can do it but you have to go through all these seemingly stupid tests where you feel so nervous and don't do as well as you could do.' Fey was convinced that she had failed therapeutics, having done a very bad paper. Will, David, Mark, Sarah, Nick and Jane seemed quietly confident that they had done enough to pass.

Dong Chiu felt everything was going well until the last day of the exams. Her clinical and viva in surgery were to be held at Wexham Park Hospital in Slough, and she travelled there by train from Paddington with a group of other students. The viva was the stuff of nightmares. Dong did not know the answers to some of the questions and then nervousness paralysed her. 'I had a mental block and couldn't find the name for an extremely common disease: osteoarthritis. I just sat there and said osteo ... osteo ... osteo, and couldn't figure out what came next. I really feel I've done myself a terrible injustice.' In her clinical exam she was caught out by the short cases: although she had read about some of conditions she was examined on, she had never seen them in a patient. She was now pessimistic about her chances of passing finals. 'I feel it may turn out to be very dreadful. I watched the examiners' expressions as I was talking to them and it was quite obvious that there were some things which I should have been able to spot very quickly and didn't. They looked disapproving. The results will be out in forty-eight hours, but I wish I knew them now.'

The morning of results day was the longest in creation. The list was to go up in the medical school at midday, but most candidates slept badly and woke early: they had hours to kill. They took long, tense breakfasts, drank countless cups of coffee, walked around Hyde Park. Time crawled. Finally they dragged themselves into the medical school and loitered in the lobby, creatures in limbo.

Will, Ese, John and Fey were the first batch of our doctors to sit finals, in June 1990. John was in Plymouth and planned to receive his results by telephone. All the others went to the medical school and watched as the list was pinned to the board.

Ese stared at the results board for an age, then grinned from ear to ear. The first thing she did was to telephone her foster mother in Chesterfield. 'Hello Mum. ... Passed.' After that Ese's end of the call consisted of much giggling and sniffing. Later, she cried with relief. Will, too, had passed, but reacted with bewildered understatement. 'It's rather an emotional moment. I can't quite believe it's all over. I'm very pleased that I can now start doing what I originally set out to do six years ago.'

Fey, who was convinced she had failed after performing badly in two papers, circled the board warily, then dived in. Success! She spotted Will and punched the air in triumph. She drove straight home where her daughter Catherine was crouching on the front doorsteps waiting for news. Fey, beaming, drew up outside the house and handed her the results in an envelope which bore the inscription 'Dr Fey Probst'. 'Mummy's a doctor,' sang Fey. 'Stop behaving like a two-year-old,' retorted Catherine.

Meanwhile John Shephard phoned the medical school, certain that he had failed. 'I said: "OK, which ones did I go down on?" and they said medicine and clinical pharmacology.' John and Debbie were preparing for a month-long climbing expedition in Pakistan and had to leave two days after the results were announced. 'It took a while to sink in,' said John as they waited to board their plane at Heathrow. 'It didn't really hit me until a day later, when I suddenly thought: five years down the drain, and it's your own fault. So I had an afternoon of failing to cope, sitting amongst the luggage, crying my eyes out.'

Twelve months later our remaining six students waited to learn their fate. This year in addition to the list posted on the board, everyone was given an envelope containing their results at the medical school office. Sarah was one of the first to arrive and ripped open her envelope with frantic concentration. No one was in any doubt about her result: 'Ye-e-es!' she roared at the top of her voice. 'It's over!' And she disappeared into a sea of hugs. Minutes later, Jane Morris appeared out of the throng, her whole body shaken with sobs of relief, and threw her arms around Sarah. They clung to one another, laughing and crying. The atmosphere was electric: the extreme solitude of waiting and worrying having been replaced by the opposite extreme of group relief and rejoicing. Everyone seemed to be shouting, screaming and crying at once and the sound reverberated off the high ceiling of the medical school foyer.

Mark and Nick arrived after the first wave of euphoria and made their way soberly through the cacophony to claim their envelopes. Their response was markedly more controlled. 'Got it!' they said, grinning. Nick conceded, 'I feel a lot better now than I did a few seconds ago. I was OK when I got up this morning, but then I went for a walk round Hyde Park and became convinced I'd failed. It's a very, very good feeling.' Both went to phone their families. 'Hello, Mother. Success,' said Nick, now laughing with happiness. At the next telephone another male student was in tears: 'Hello, Dad, I'm a doctor. I can't stop crying, it's bloody stupid. ...' Mark stayed cool as he phoned his home: 'Mum? It's Dr George calling from Paddington here,' then began to giggle hysterically.

David Copping came with his wife to pick up his results. He too had passed. More hugs and smiles of relief. Then Dong Chiu arrived, her face a mask of apprehension. She walked slowly and deliberately to the desk and gave her name. As she opened the envelope her face exploded into a radiant smile. 'I passed all of it. I had prepared myself to expect the worst because my surgery clinicals were absolutely terrible.' She scrutinised her piece of paper again – 'just to make sure my little eyes haven't deceived me.'

Everyone headed for the basement of the medical school for a champagne reception. They took innumerable photographs of one another – group shots, embraces and close ups of the precious pieces of paper that informed them they could now put MB BS (Lond) after their names and the magic prefix 'Dr' before them. Afterwards they split into smaller groups and went back to flats and bedsits for parties which continued long into the following day.

After a weekend of drinking and celebration, the newly-qualified doctors had to endure another morning of suspense. On Monday afternoon at two o'clock the list of house jobs was posted on the medical school noticeboard. In a re-run of results day, students who had applied for jobs on the St Mary's scheme gathered round to discover where they would spend the next six months. Fey and Ese were pleased that they had both been allocated jobs at St Charles's. A year later Jane and Dong both secured their first-choice jobs, split between St Mary's and St Charles's; Mark got the post he wanted at St Mary's; and David discovered to his relief that he had been allocated one of his chosen jobs close to home. Nick had failed to get the top medicine job at St Mary's that he had put first, but was pleased to have secured a surgical post in Slough. Sarah, who had planned to do a medical job first, was amazed to find she had been allocated to the academic surgical unit at St Mary's since she had put the job last on her list, after six medical ones.

Now there was nothing to keep them in London and, with five weeks before they started work as house officers there was a lot of unwinding to be done. Many went away with their parents on a final, celebratory family holiday. It was the end of five or six years of emotional and financial support. The parents of students who received only the minimum government grants had invested huge sums in their children's education: estimates varied between £20 000 and £50 000. In addition, most students had substantial overdrafts by the time they graduated and a small number owed their banks more than £10 000.

Two months after failing finals, John Shephard was aboard a car ferry sailing the Plymouth-Jersey route. John was working as Chief Relief Officer, which brought a much-needed £50 a day into the Shephard coffers. Ironically, the exam results had come out on Debbie's last day at work: she had left her estate agent's office after six years of supporting John in order to return to college herself and she was now training to become a teacher. Her career change had been based on the assumption that John would be earning a houseman's salary in the autumn; as it turned out he was still on a grant and had to work to supplement their income. John was now philosophical about his finals failure. 'Failing is not something anyone would want to do, but I have learned a lot as a result. I have had two months to stop and think, which is not normally possible in a medical training. I have realised that medicine is not the centre of the universe.'

University of London regulations meant that John had to do another three months' work before retaking his exams. He spent three days a week on the wards at the Central Middlesex Hospital and the rest of his time on book work. By December, when he sat his retakes, John felt better prepared – he had read much more widely and had concentrated on areas where he knew he was weak – but he nevertheless felt terribly nervous. 'It's harder the second time round because you know what's coming and there's a lot more hanging on it. Failing once is not a disaster, failing twice is stupidity and would be very damaging to one's ego.'

As John sat his final exam, Debbie waited on tenterhooks in the Medical School. 'It will be nice to get it over with, whichever way it goes,' she commented. 'The pressure is immense.' Half an hour after the exam ended, John, Debbie and a handful of other re-sit candidates paced the foyer of the medical school waiting for the results list to go up. As the paper was pinned to the board, John moved forward like a man at the scaffold, Debbie hovering nervously behind him. Then he turned, beaming, and swung her off her feet, announcing in disbelief, 'I've passed.' His first action was to run across Praed Street to the nearest off-licence and he returned to the medical school bearing a bottle of Bollinger. As they sipped champagne he and Debbie smiled and laughed with relief.

John said that failure had been a bruising experience – but had taught him a great deal. 'I feel I've paid quite a price for failing, but I think I'll make a better doctor now. During the last couple of weeks I couldn't stand being on my own any longer which is why Debbie is here today. I've realised I'm vulnerable myself, and as a result I think I'm now more compassionate.' John now looked forward to two months off, climbing in Scotland, before starting work in Torquay in February. Debbie looked forward to having her husband at home. 'Now we can play at being married at last.'

8

DOCTORS AT LAST

No doctor ever forgets his or her first day as a house officer on the wards. Talk to the most illustrious surgeons or physicians and they will describe the excitement, anxiety and confusion of that first twenty-four hours as qualified doctors. After five or six years of being lectured and hectored, of observing and shadowing, they are finally given real responsibility. They have patients of their own. They write prescriptions for drugs. They are called to see emergency cases in casualty and have to decide quickly and correctly what is wrong and what treatment must be given. The long rehearsal is over and the performance has begun.

House officers are at the bottom of the medical pile, junior members of the firm; but they are crucial to its smooth functioning. They have the greatest contact with patients, spending most of their time on the wards, talking, examining, assessing, ordering tests and liaising with nurses, social workers, laboratories and patients' families. They are the foot-soldiers of the firm; if they fail to do their work with skill and efficiency, patients suffer and the whole enterprise can grind to a halt.

August 1 is always a chaotic and stressful day in hospitals throughout the country. Thousands of house officers, SHOs and registrars change jobs simultaneously on this day and often only one or two people on a firm are familiar with the hospital, the staff and the patients. For this reason, doctors often joke that it is better to suffer agonies rather than go anywhere near a hospital on the first day of August. The new house officers are almost always thrown in at the deep end. They may have attended an induction session the previous day when they will have been introduced to their hospital and given basic information about administration and support services. They may even have met their predecessors for a hand-over of patients and advice. But nothing prepares them for their first real taste of medical responsibility. Our students, like all the others, arrived between 7.30 and 8 A.M., bursting with excitement and apprehension. The pale-faced undergraduates who grappled with final exams had metamorphosed into sleek, suntanned young professionals during their five-week break since results day. Most had spent the interlude on Mediterranean beaches, basking in that first, sweetest, phase of a medical career, when their new status was unsullied by its attendant burdens and responsibilities. Clothes, often bought specially in anticipation of the first professional pay packet, were smart and stylish.

The first port of call was the laundry, where full-length white coats lay in piles. For the first time they pulled on this uniform of office, luxurious after three years of the abbreviated student version, and attached their new name badges. Brand new notebooks and Filofaxes were slipped into pockets, then they headed for the hospital switchboard to collect their bleeps and keys to the rooms in the hospital where they would sleep when on call. Suitably equipped, they tried to make contact with their firms. This was often difficult. Their first point of contact would normally be the SHOs, but, likely as not, they too were new to the hospital, and knew nothing about the firm's schedule. If the new doctors were lucky, a sympathetic and knowledgeable senior would spot their plight and provide a rapid, pragmatic introduction to the firm. If not, they could flounder for days.

Most unfortunate were the house officers who found themselves 'on take' on their first day. Firms took it in turns to handle emergency admissions who came into casualty or were referred to hospital by general practitioners. They were on call for twenty-four-hour stints during the week and for periods of up to seventy-two hours over weekends. Some firms were on take one day in every nine (known as 'a one in nine'). Busier firms could work a one in three rota – and when one member of the team was ill or on leave, this might turn into a one in two where every other day and night were spent working in the hospital.

Sarah Holdsworth confessed that she was dreading her first day as an orthopaedic house officer at St Mary's. She did not want to make a career in surgery and the job, rumoured to be a tough one, had been her last choice. Sarah was scared that her natural forgetfulness would lead to terrible errors: she wondered whether she would cope at all. The discovery that she was on take on August 1 increased her anxiety. As she walked to the hospital along streets bathed in early morning sunshine in her new floral-patterned dress and sensible shoes she prayed that she would not be simply left to cope on her own. Her prayer went unanswered.

Sarah's consultant was on holiday. Her senior registrar was busy seeing patients in the fracture clinic. Her SHO was based at St Charles's Hospital, two miles away, during the daytime. So when the first orthopaedic patient came into casualty, Sarah was the only doctor left to bleep. She was told that a man had fallen out of a fourth floor window and fractured his pelvis. Arriving in casualty, she discovered that the story was more complicated. David, aged forty-two, had jumped from his window in an attempt to commit suicide, but landed on a roof, injuring his spine and pelvis. He told her that his girlfriend had taken an overdose the previous week and died in St Mary's. He could not face life without her, but had not managed to kill himself. He had been a heroin addict for twenty years: please could Sarah prescribe him some methadone (a heroin substitute), because he was getting withdrawal symptoms?

Sarah had never encountered a drug abuser before; she had never dealt with a suicide attempt; and she had never seen a fractured pelvis, although she knew that it was a potentially dangerous condition that could result in internal injuries. The patient might bleed to death.

First she had to clerk the patient. This was difficult because he was wearing an oxygen mask which muffled his voice. She then had to examine him: fortunately he showed no signs of paralysis – always a risk with spinal injuries – but any movement of his lower trunk and legs was excruciatingly painful. Sarah knew she had to roll him over in order to examine his back, but had no idea how to do it. Eventually she found a young nurse to help her and together they managed to bundle a screaming David on to his side. Sarah confessed afterwards, 'I didn't get much assistance and I would have liked a bit more support – it was a nightmare. Medical school didn't prepare me for this!'

Much later, after David had been admitted to one of the wards, Sarah had a chance to ask one of the consultants for advice. She explained that her patient was a registered heroin addict who wanted her to prescribe him some methadone. She didn't know whether she was allowed to because it was a dangerous drug: what should she do? The consultant smiled at her anxiety. 'Give him some: you're the one in the driving seat now.'

At St Charles's Hospital, Jane Morris was working for a firm of general surgeons and, like Sarah, found herself having to tackle difficult situations alone. She spent most of her first day looking after an eighty-four-year-old woman who had just had a major operation to remove a tumour from her oesophagus. She was now on a ventilator to maintain her breathing and needed constant monitoring. Jane had been told that the woman was the most seriously ill patient in the hospital, and, as the most junior member of the firm, she was terrified by the responsibility. She tried to bleep her seniors, but they did not respond. Their bleeps, she found out later, were broken.

Jane was better able to cope with the demands of her first day than some of her colleagues because both the hospital and the team were familiar. She had spent a total of three months on the firm while studying surgery as a clinical student and had also done a student assistantship or 'locum' there. Students had an opportunity to work as locums while house officers took holidays. They were not allowed to prescribe drugs or to prepare patients for theatre, but they carried bleeps, slept in the hospital when on take, and looked after in-patients. Locums typically lasted for two weeks and gave final-year medical students an invaluable insight into the life of a qualified doctor. They soon gleaned nuggets of information that were vital for survival: the whereabouts of the pathology laboratory where they had to take blood for testing, the quickest way from the wards to casualty, the idiosyncrasies of consultants and ward sisters and the opening hours of the canteen.

For many new house officers, simple procedures like taking blood or putting in drips could turn into an ordeal. Their three years of clinical medicine had given them opportunities to practise the techniques, but there was always someone on hand to take over if things went wrong. Now they had to take blood quickly and efficiently from all patients, including the ones with 'no veins' from whom they had been protected as students. These included very elderly patients whose blood vessels had collapsed, emergency admissions whose circulation had 'shut down' in response to a serious injury and long-stay patients whose veins had been damaged by repeated injections. During the first few weeks many patients suffered heroically at the trembling hands of their inexperienced doctors.

Dong Chiu and Mark George, who were both with surgical firms at St Mary's, each encountered difficulties. Dong had five attempts at taking blood from one woman, and spilt so much in the process that the sheets had to be changed afterwards. Mark, who had acquired such a reputation for inept blood-taking as a student that the bruises he caused were widely known as Georgeomas (the medical term for a bruise is haematoma), generally needed several stabs at a vein before he hit his target. He admitted he had a problem putting in drips. 'I can't work it out: I seem to get the needle into the vein, then it comes out again. It's a bit depressing – every time I hear I've got to put one in I think, "Poor patient, here's another four or five attempts!" ' Neither Mark nor Dong was unusual: none of the house officers had had sufficient practical experience as a student, so they had to learn while doing the job. Patients were, in general, oblivious of this fact and one rookie houseman recounted to roars of laughter how a woman in the private Lindo Wing at St Mary's had declined the services of the phlebotomist (a professional and expert blood-taker) insisting that a 'qualified doctor' must take her blood. He went to see her and spent twenty minutes repeatedly puncturing her forearm before he struck blood.

Intravenous drug abusers were notoriously difficult subjects when it came to taking blood or putting up drips. Their drug habit often meant that almost all their veins had collapsed and there was nowhere left to inject. Often the only solution was to ask them to insert the needle themselves (practice having made them far more proficient than a new house officer) or to cut into the skin in search of a deeper, healthier vein. Paddington had a large population of drug addicts and during her first week Sarah Holdsworth admitted five through casualty. After the initial shock of coping with David, she learned how to deal with them. 'At first I felt really embarrassed about bringing the subject up and getting them to talk about their drug habit. I didn't know what to say or what questions to ask. I was afraid I'd sound patronising if I asked them why they did it. Now I'm used to it and I ask them whether they go to needle exchanges or a drug dependence unit and whether they have ever thought of trying to come off.'

Like many of her colleagues, Sarah was frightened of catching HIV, the AIDS virus, from patients who injected drugs. An estimated 1 in every 250 people in the Paddington area were HIV positive and doctors were exposed to infection when they took blood or operated on such patients. David, her first patient, was aware of the risks he ran and had had an HIV test several months earlier which had proved negative. He was happy to talk about the issue to Sarah (and to be filmed doing so) and he agreed when she suggested he should have another test. Other patients were less open, and so medical staff frequently had to take measures to protect themselves. When a patient thought to be high-risk for HIV or hepatitis was admitted to hospital, doctors were advised to wear gloves while taking blood or doing any other invasive procedures. Similarly, when a high-risk patient needed surgery, the operating theatre was cleared of everything but essential equipment, and surgeons wore two pairs of gloves, rubber boots and special perspex visors or goggles to protect their eyes and skin from infected blood which might spurt into their faces.

For Will Liddell the Royal United Hospital in Bath was uncharted territory. He was the most junior member of a very busy surgical firm and on his first day had to try to make sense of a sprawling district general hospital and introduce himself to the patients for whom he was now directly responsible. He was helped by a friendly senior house officer who joined him for breakfast on

August 1 and set out a few ground rules and tips for survival. Some were practical: 'Take advice from the nursing staff – most of them have been here a long time. They may not be right, but they are more likely to be right than you to start with. If one of the senior nurses says, "I think you're out of your depth, call the registrar," then do so.' Others were political: 'If a GP phones up and wants to send a patient in to you, don't refuse to take the referral. Half the GPs play golf with our bosses and that's where the bosses get their private practice – you have to watch it a bit!'

Unlike many surgical housemen, Will was seldom expected to take part in operations. While the rest of the firm were in theatre, or in out-patient clinics, he took care of all the ward work, getting to know and supervising the day-to-day care of between thirty and forty patients. The work was exhausting: Will had to take scores of blood samples and put in dozens of intravenous drips, and everywhere he went there were piles of drug charts to fill in, letters to write and discharge forms to complete. Every task seemed to be interrupted by the peevish call of his bleep as nurses, senior doctors, labs and GPs demanded his attention. For the clinical student deputising for a qualified doctor, the bleep had been a blissful symbol of power and status. Once a houseman, it quickly became a hated companion that crouched in the pocket, constantly poised to scream, preventing the orderly completion of duties. By night it was the shrill harbinger of sleeplessness.

Will was on take on his second day. He had not been taken on a tour of the hospital and was still unfamiliar with its geography and organisation. The first time his bleep went off summoning him to casualty he got lost and had to ask the attendant camera crew for directions. He was on take for a total of seventy-two hours during his first five days and got very little sleep. Several of his patients were seriously ill and he immediately became involved in their emotional as well as medical support.

One was a seventy-one-year-old man who had been admitted to hospital two days before Will arrived with pain in one of his legs. A blood clot in an artery in his thigh had stopped the circulation in his leg and he was given drugs designed to disperse the blockage. But they failed to work and on Will's third day, with the leg now numb and ice-cold, the consultant told the patient bluntly, 'I think that's going to have to come off over this weekend. OK?' It fell to Will to prepare him for the operating theatre and to talk to him about what the amputation would involve and how he would cope afterwards.

Will was unhappy that he had not established a better rapport with the man, who was delirious as a result of an infection that had developed in his leg. 'He was already on the ward when I started this job and I haven't got him to tell me how he feels about losing his leg, although he quite clearly feels awful about it. I haven't developed enough skills in talking to people about this kind of problem yet and I feel rather inadequate. I would have like to have made better friends with him before this operation so that afterwards I could be more supportive. I have prepared him for theatre physically, but not emotionally.'

Another patient, fifty-eight-year-old Mr Gedge, had already been in hospital for three weeks. He had come in for investigations on a small innocuous-looking lump on his neck, but the lump had grown rapidly and the surgeons had been unable to find a cause. After the ward round on his first day, Will was asked to arrange an urgent body scan. When the results were obtained the following day they showed a large, inoperable tumour and the prognosis was appalling: Mr Gedge had just a few days to live. The nurses broke the news to him, then Will went to see him to discuss the implications. They talked about the details of Mr Gedge's will and about his diagnosis. 'I know the worst, and there's nothing we can do about it: I've just got to take things hour by hour from now on,' said Mr Gedge.

'I think we talked reasonably directly,' Will said afterwards. 'There is a terrible temptation when you're having a conversation about the fact that someone is about to die to talk in euphemisms and skirt around the subject and you can end up having a terrible non-conversation, but I think that Mr Gedge now understands the nature of his disease. I really hope that he has a bit more than a few days, so that he and his wife can talk about it properly.'

Will regretted that medical school had not taught him the skill of breaking bad news. 'This is not something which you *have* to learn in a live situation on a real person: you can and should rehearse it. The moment when you're told that your husband has only a few weeks to live must be one of the most devastating moments of a person's life and anything that can be done to make it easier by proper training of the people giving the news is well worth it. Probably the most important thing you can learn to do for patients is to counsel their relatives.'

In his first few days Will had faced the kind of emotional challenges that most newly qualified doctors dread. Several of his patients were terminally ill and he felt drained. Then, three days after he started at Bath, news came from St Mary's that two close friends from the medical school had been killed while climbing in Kenya with a St Mary's Mountaineering Club expedition that Will himself had originally hoped to join. Speaking about the tragedy after fourteen hours on call, Will looked exhausted and was close to tears, but he felt that the experience had brought him closer to the suffering of some of his patients and their families. 'You would have to multiply what I feel about my friends several times to reach the level of regret that will be experienced by Mrs Gedge and the spouses of the other terminally ill people in my care. In small measure I know something of the dreadful emptiness they will feel.'

Although our doctors had already spent three years on the wards, many of them seemed to encounter the tough aspects of medicine for the first time as house officers. This was partly because they had been protected from 'difficult' cases while they were students, and because trainee doctors were not expected to grapple with drunk, drugged, angry or hysterical patients. Now they were expected to cope with everything. During her first on-take weekend, ten days into the job and already noticeably more confident and competent, Sarah was called to casualty to see a young woman. She was a typical weekend visitor to the busy Paddington accident and emergency department, but Sarah had not encountered her like before. Cheryl was a pretty, lively twenty-five-year-old in a tight red mini dress and inadequate shoes who was very, very drunk. She had spent Saturday morning drinking with friends, then lurched back to her room over the road from St Mary's to make lunch – and had sliced open her little finger with a vegetable knife, severing a tendon and a nerve. Now she sat giggling in a casualty examination room, the gashed finger drooping disobediently as she held out her hand, palm uppermost, and told Sarah the story.

It was difficult to obtain a straightforward medical history from Cheryl. Her replies constantly went off at a tangent and her boyfriend kept interrupting. When Sarah told her she would have to come into hospital to have her finger repaired under general anaesthetic, Cheryl burst into tears and cried noisily for several minutes. 'You didn't tell me I had to have an operation. I didn't think it was that bad,' she shouted accusingly. 'I hate hospitals and what am I going to do with my little boy – he's only two? Why can't you just stick a needle in and do it right now?'

Sarah explained as patiently as she could that the injury was too serious to be treated under local anaesthetic, but she left the consultation reeling from the encounter. 'I'm having a nightmare,' she said to her SHO. 'And she's having hysterics.' She had to arrange a bed and book an operating theatre for that evening. In the event, the anaesthetist discovered that Cheryl had grown thirsty in casualty and consumed yet another pint of beer after Sarah had seen her. As a result she still had too much alcohol in her blood to undergo surgery safely and the operation had to be postponed until the following morning.

The operation was a success and soon afterwards Sarah told Cheryl that she could go home. Now sober and much quieter, Cheryl said goodbye. 'Thank you for everything you've done for me, doctor. I couldn't have gone through it without you. You was me inspiration with all them needles.' Sarah said that dealing with Cheryl had been rewarding, despite her tantrums and demands. 'I think I made her see a bit of sense. And even though she's from a completely different background from me, we did manage to make some kind of relationship. Our lives touched for a short time, and I think I helped her.'

The opportunity to perform practical procedures, particularly in surgery, also brought rewards. Jane Morris glowed with pleasure after removing a collection of cysts and swellings from the heads and necks of four patients who came in on her second day. It was 'day case' surgery – minor stuff done under local anaesthetic, but new territory for Jane. 'It's good to be *doing* something as opposed to just taking bloods and filling in forms,' she said afterwards. 'We couldn't really do this kind of thing before now: people are a bit unwilling to have a medical student digging around in their necks, but oddly enough, once you're qualified, they will let you do anything!'

Fey Probst, working with the Dean's medical firm at St Charles's, revelled in her encounters with patients. Of all our new doctors, Fey was the most outspoken and ecstatic about the pleasures of medicine. She was friendly, sympathetic and protective towards her patients, and keen to be involved whenever an extra pair of hands seemed to be needed. At 2 A.M. on Sunday during her first weekend on call she was making her way to her room in the hospital, having checked that all was well with her patients on the wards. As she passed the entrance to casualty, she noticed a flurry of activity and discovered that ten people had just come in with serious injuries.

Fey offered to help and spent the next four hours helping the surgeons stabilise the patients. The following morning she was exhausted, but there was a full day's work to be done, and by the time Peter Richards came to the hospital for his Sunday evening ward round at nine o'clock, Fey's chalk-white face and hollow eyes bore witness to her lack of sleep. Professor Richards asked how she had coped with her first on-take weekend and she replied with a colourful account of the nocturnal emergency. When it became clear that the patients in question had not belonged to his firm and had been surgical rather than medical, Peter Richards had a gentle word with Fey's registrar Dr Levin David, who told her, 'The Prof is highly appreciative of your performance, but he feels you need to survive your twelve months as a house officer. If you go looking for work, medicine will become a twenty-four-hour business. The best way to survive is to confine yourself to your own patients. So tonight, get some sleep!' And, to ensure that she did, Dr David took Fey's on-call bleep and answered it for her during the night.

Fey, with her four children, her au pairs and her ramshackle house in distant Bow, had been out of the ordinary as a medical student. She was an equally eccentric house officer. By the time she finished medical school, she was £13 000 in debt, yet, in anticipation of her first pay packet, she had spent £5000 on a shiny new 650cc motorbike, capable of doing 160mph. Every day she roared the eight miles from Bow to Notting Hill clad in bicycle leathers and helmet and changed into a blouse and skirt in her hospital room. On the days when she wasn't on call, she aimed to get home by 5.30 P.M. and spent her evenings supervising the children's homework, cooking supper and trying to catch up on the ironing. She was perpetually on the run, yet radiated happiness. 'I have never had a moment's regret about entering medicine,' she commented at the end of her house officer year. 'It has been well worth it and I am having a marvellous time.'

Not all new house officers found relating to patients so easy. Some went to the opposite extreme, often performing complex and painful procedures that lasted many minutes without addressing a single word to the patient. Experienced ward sisters confirmed that such behaviour was not uncommon: some house officers did not begin to talk to patients for months. They seemed so absorbed in and anxious about the technical aspects of the job in hand that they had nothing to spare for the human being at the end of the stethoscope or syringe. Part of the problem was undoubtedly the volume of work they had to get through – particularly at the beginning when they had not yet evolved an efficient system of personal record keeping or learned how best to organise their days. Many appeared to regard patients as obstacles in an assault course, to be approached with wary determination and got past as quickly as possible so that one more name could be crossed off the unending list. Even those who were basically comfortable with patients complained that there simply was not time to get to know them in the way they had hoped. Nick Hollings summed the problem up succinctly when he explained his strategy for efficient communication: he asked patients if they had any questions, but put it in such a way that they had to answer no.

John Shephard started his house job at Torbay District General Hospital on 1 February 1991. The Gulf War was about to begin and the former Merchant Navy officer suffered a twinge of nostalgia on his first morning as he walked past the stall in the hospital entrance collecting gifts and money for servicemen. 'Part of me wants to be part of the action, putting into practice the things I was trained to do,' he said. Instead, John found himself

on the surgical front line. He had come to join the urology firm –
a specialist team which dealt with diseases and disorders affecting
the kidneys, urinary tract and bladder. Today the firm was on
call and he would see all surgical patients admitted to the hospital.

John had a brief meeting with his consultant, Mr Richard
Bradbrook, who then left to deal with patients at another hospital
eight miles away. The senior registrar greeted John, then disappeared into the operating theatre for a morning of surgery.
The only remaining member of the firm was John's immediate
superior, a shy Indian SHO who had arrived in Britain for the
first time three days earlier. Almost immediately John's bleep
went off and he spent the next five hours in casualty, dealing on
his own with patient after patient. There was a lull in the afternoon when he managed to visit the three wards where the firm
had patients to do routine work such as taking blood, giving drugs
and catching up with paperwork. Then he was called to casualty
again and worked right through the evening.

At one o'clock in the morning, he had to assist the senior
registrar in a difficult procedure: a young man had been admitted
in agony, having been unable to pass urine for more than twenty-
four hours. Rather than pass a tube into his penis, the team
decided to relieve the pressure by giving him a local anaesthetic,
then pushing a plastic tube through the man's abdominal wall and
into his overstretched bladder to release the urine. Immediately
afterwards, John was called to the operating theatre to assist at
an emergency operation on an elderly lady with a life-threatening
abdominal emergency. He spent four hours in theatre and fell
asleep at the operating table. He went to bed at 6.30 A.M. and
was up again at 8.15 A.M. to take part in a ward round.

His first twenty-two hours in the job were 'a bit of a baptism
of fire', he said, but his years in the navy had prepared him for
long hours and little sleep. He admitted that he did not feel
qualified to do the job and sometimes had no idea what to do.
'There's a lot of front. But you have to appear confident, otherwise
you're lost: the patients will smell it and they won't take you
seriously.'

After five or six years on a student grant, all our doctors were relieved to be earning at last, and derived much pleasure from speculating how they would spend their first salary cheques. Sarah wanted to save up for her first car and buy some hi-fi equipment. Nick was keen to trade in his current vehicle for something longer and lower, but for the first two years that would be out of the question: he was paying off his overdraft at the rate of £450 a month. Most house officers lived in shared houses with low rents or in heavily-subsidised hospital accommodation and they saw their first year as doctors as an opportunity to earn a reasonable salary while living very cheaply.

In 1991 the average basic salary was £12 100, but could be pushed up to £17 000 by the colossal amounts of overtime worked by house officers. The pay for the additional hours was *one third* of the basic hourly rate – an exploitation of captive professional labour which provoked anger and bitterness among junior doctors and generally met with disbelief among non-medics. These over-time rates made house officers the cheapest people employed in the hospital after 5 P.M. The justification for the low payment used to be that during their on-call periods hospital doctors, though required to be on the premises, might well have nothing to do. In practice, according to a report in 1989, most house officers in teaching hospitals were actually working for 75 hours of the 140 they were theoretically on call. During weeks when they did an on-take weekend, the hours they were actually at work rose to 124.

Our ten doctors were interviewed about their pay and con-ditions during their first weeks as house officers. They all criticised the system, but most seemed resigned to making the best of a bad year. They said they had always known that the house jobs would be hard, allowing little time for a social life or even sleep. All had discovered that house officers were the lowest form of medical life and could do little right. Jane redefined the job. 'You're a cross between a porter and a clerk.' And Sarah listed the qualities she now considered essential in her work. 'You mustn't be very sensitive, otherwise you wouldn't cope with all the work they pile on to you, and you have to be tough. And you have to realise that everyone will blame you.' Almost everyone complained about this. It was the house officer's job to keep notes up to date and to ensure that all test results, X-rays and letters were constantly to hand. No matter who had spirited away the patient's file or some vital piece of paper, when a senior doctor looked in vain for it, it was *always* the houseman's fault.

Jane's marriage was eight months away. She and her fiancé Tony Gilbert confessed that the pressures of Jane's job were already telling: tiredness was making her bad tempered and easily upset and they realised that Jane's hours would mean they had much less time together. They had already begun to compare diaries weeks in advance in order to guarantee an evening together. Like many female junior doctors, Jane was concerned about combining a medical career with marriage and children. She hoped to become a gynaecologist and would therefore have to scale the surgical ladder, a fiercely competitive career path, designed by men for men, which made little allowance for child-bearing and rearing.

Sarah, too, worried about the future. After two weeks she felt exhausted and wondered how she would manage for a year. She was also concerned about her relationship with her boyfriend of five years, who was also a sailing partner. She felt that the pay was too low, mainly because a basic salary of £12 000 did not sufficiently compensate junior doctors against the increasing risk of HIV infection. Her satisfaction in the work was tempered by a sense of loss. 'It's like throwing away another part of your childhood. You can't shrink behind other people any more, you have finally to take responsibility and make decisions. It's tough.'

Not everyone was pessimistic about the job. David Copping was working with a medical firm at the Central Middlesex Hospital in Park Royal, west London. He had a light on-take rota, and felt well supported by senior members of his team. 'I have plenty of time to sit down and talk to patients. I don't feel overworked and I have no regrets about entering medicine.' At St Mary's, Mark George was equally happy, 'I've settled down and I'm quite enjoying myself. I'm with a good team and I'm getting lots of teaching. When we have a busy on-take night I do feel very tired the following evening, but the whole job is still quite a novel experience – so far I've got no regrets.' Dong Chiu felt that she was managing, though the job occupied all her time. 'I have done nothing but work, come home and go to sleep for six weeks and I can't go on like this. I shall become very dull and boring!'

At the beginning of the house officer year the excitement and euphoria of working as qualified doctors buoyed the spirits of our group and they were glad to be practising at last. Several months into their jobs, the first four to qualify – Ese, Will, Fey and John – had very different attitudes and opinions. At the end of his house jobs, Will reflected that it had been an extraordinary year. 'The privations, abuses, frequent loss of temper and frustration have been amazing, but I *seem* to have enjoyed it nevertheless. The main bonus has been friendships – very intense ones – nurtured by the shared horrors of housemanship.' Will planned to return to the West Country to embark upon a two-and-a-half-year GP training scheme based in Bath.

Ese now seemed to hate medicine. 'It's a dog's life. If I could get out and do something else, I would. If someone had shown me at eighteen what a house officer does, I wouldn't have applied to medical school.' Ese, who was now working on a very busy medical firm at St Mary's, described endless broken nights and the horror of trying to get through a demanding day's work after two or three hours' sleep. 'Finals weren't even painful compared with this: this is torture. All you think about is eating and getting enough sleep. When you get bleeped in the middle of the night, you try not to wake up completely, otherwise you're wide awake when you get back to bed and cannot get off to sleep. I've sometimes clerked and prescribed drugs for patients in the middle of the night, and the following morning, although my handwriting is in their notes, I haven't been able to remember anything about it at all.'

Her firm tended to deal with seriously ill patients, many of them dying of liver failure, and Ese had often found herself handling medical emergencies alone. Several of her patients had died and she had drawn on her strong Christian faith to make sense of what was happening and to comfort relatives. She felt that she had a contribution to make and still loved working with patients, but the personal sacrifices demanded by the job were simply too great. Halfway through her house officer year Ese and Simon Stacey, her boyfriend during most of the years at medical school, decided to get married. The wedding took place in October 1991 and Ese decided to leave medicine for a year in order to take stock of her career. She had already shelved plans to qualify as a surgeon because of the total commitment and long hours demanded in the specialty. She wanted to take up athletics again – training had been impossible during most of her house year – and work out what to do next. In the meantime, she enrolled for courses in French, Portuguese and computing. Ese reported that morale was low among many of her colleagues: doctors at St Mary's right up to senior registrar level could be heard wondering aloud whether they had been right to enter medicine.

Four months into his first house job, John Shephard was deeply disillusioned. He found the work brutalising, the hours long and the rewards inadequate. He too confessed that, if he had known what life as a junior doctor would be like, he would not have left the navy to go to medical school. And he revealed that the stress of the job was seriously affecting his relationship with his wife Debbie. He felt very close to the doctors and nurses he worked with: they shared the burdens and understood the strains, and when he finally arrived home, he didn't want to speak to anyone. He had used up all his compassion, concern and interest in other people and he simply wanted to be alone. 'This isn't a job for a married man,' he said. 'If you are in your early twenties, it's OK: when the work is finished, you can all go off and get drunk together, or all go sailing.'

Debbie, who had provided emotional and financial support throughout John's time at St Mary's, was now desperately worried about his job and the effects it was having upon their marriage. She had survived five years of separation, had propped him up during the previous summer when he had failed finals, and had looked forward to John's first job, when they would be able to live together again. In the event, she saw less of him than before, and he was perpetually tired. She said that he had lost weight and aged considerably during his first four months, and he no longer had any time for her. 'John has always been a very caring person, and he still is – but now all his caring goes to the patients and there is none left for me.' Debbie was unsure whether their marriage would survive the pressures being put on them by medicine. John had recently told her that he had to decide whether to train to be a GP and stay with her or to do surgery and divorce her.

In August John began his second house job at Derriford Hospital, Plymouth, a ten-minute bike ride from his home. He had shed the horrors of commuting, but the punishing hours continued – and for the first time he began seriously to contemplate giving up medicine. 'This is much harder than being at sea. I have never worked so hard, so continuously in my life. The whole system is wrong: I have worked very hard for virtually no reward. This job destroys you and the concept of just walking away from it is extremely appealing.' His long-term ambition was still to become a surgeon and he talked of the jobs he would apply for next in order to begin training for a surgical career, but he spoke of surgery as an addiction. 'It's like heroin: you'd give it up if you could but you're hooked.'

During August 1991, John worked 320 hours and earned £900. He worked twenty-nine days and had two off. 'I love medicine, but I loathe the job conditions,' he said. 'They degrade and brutalise you and make absolutely no allowance for the fact that you're a human being. I started to feel like this after about six weeks. Initially it was exciting to be a doctor at last but the job is making my marriage almost impossible. By the time I get home I have given all day and haven't got anything left. I either want to be left totally on my own or just go to bed. If I'd known what medicine was going to be like before I applied six years ago, I wouldn't have touched it. It could have been such a wonderful thing to be a doctor but it's not, it's a disaster. The system stinks. There are too many whitewashes in medicine. It's time people knew what they are doing to doctors.'

Debbie felt angry at the treatment of junior hospital doctors. 'They're talking about cutting the hours to seventy-two per week; but that's twice what the Ford workers are asking for, and which is more important, building motor cars or mending people? There is not enough thought put into caring for the people who are doing the caring and it makes me very cross to see the way they are overworked, they're drained, and nobody cares about them.

I hate the system for what it's doing to John. I was looking forward to having him home and having fun. Actually we're spending less time together than when John was a medical student in London. It's unbelievable to watch someone change so much in such a short time.'

What went wrong? All our students entered medical school bursting with enthusiasm and a desire to do good. They trained for five years at considerable cost to the taxpayer and were proud and pleased to enter the profession. Within a few months quite a few had become cynical, bitter and very angry. Two of them are actively considering abandoning medicine. They were not unusual: many of their peers were also profoundly disillusioned.

After six weeks on the wards, Jane, for example, was enjoying the work, but had some very bad days when she had doubts about her choice of career. 'I don't know whether I'd do it again. I hadn't anticipated such long hours for so little pay for so long. I thought about it in my final year, but over the last couple of weeks, the thought of doing this for forty years is terrible. It has put me off hospital medicine a lot. I feel angry about the conditions that we have to work. Tony, my fiancé, has a great lifestyle doing law and he and his colleagues are no more intelligent or better qualified than us. He earns more than twice as much as my salary, including overtime. It would be a great job if you were just doing the medicine and seeing patients, but seventy per cent of my time is spent chasing test results, organising theatre lists and taking blood.'

There were many reasons for their discontent. In 1984 when they applied to medical school they saw medicine as a demanding but socially useful and rewarding job. They knew that the training was long and that junior doctors worked unsocial hours (though most of those interviewed substantially underestimated the number of hours) but they believed that at the end of the training a good salary and high status would be theirs. Most of them were supported by parents who saw medicine as an excellent career option and were proud to have sons and daughters at medical school.

But during the late 1980s public perceptions of the medical profession would begin to change. Junior hospital doctors complained increasingly loudly about their conditions, pointing out that an average working week of ninety hours was hardly conducive to patient safety, let alone high quality of care. There were threats of strikes, and reports in the medical press suggesting that many young doctors were voting with their feet and leaving the profession. A survey published in 1988, when our ten were in the midst of their clinical studies, found that among a large group of doctors who had qualified in 1981, almost half regretted they had chosen a career in medicine. The survey's author, Isobel Allen, commented, 'When I started this research, I was not prepared for the welter of depression and pessimism which greeted any question about career opportunities or future prospects. Many of the young doctors said their original decision to enter medical school was based on myth rather than reality. When they qualified, many were devastated by the pre-registration year.' Allen says some responses to her questionnaire read like suicide notes.

Nick Hollings, doing surgery at Wexham Park Hospital in Slough, was not suicidal, but he was disillusioned. 'The pay is appalling and it's a real source of anger, especially at weekends, when you look at the cleaners and know they are getting paid more than we are as house officers.'

'At the moment, I feel that it's an all right job, but nothing more. I know it will get better: the amount of donkey work will drop. But I am still not sufficiently convinced to see it as my career for the rest of my life. Once, at four o'clock in the morning, after a weekend when I had had seven hours' sleep in a fifty-six-hour period on call, I gave twice the appropriate dose of drug because I was so tired. Fortunately the patient did not suffer, but he could have done: the mistake was the result of complete exhaustion.

'Medical school did not prepare me for the sheer drudgery of seventy-five per cent of the work and the terrible stress of the first week. Suddenly you're qualified and terrified of not asking a patient the right questions and them dying as a result. It is very worrying indeed. You just don't know what you are doing. I got through it by saying to myself, "Come on, mate, don't be pathetic, you can do this."'

Nick felt that medical school could have prepared him better for dealing with death. Four patients died during his first six weeks and he found the experience gruelling. 'I have had to comfort relatives and I am still very green. Even now after four times, I find it very difficult. It's always the poor housedog who has to do it and I would have liked to do some role-playing with actors at medical school or watch house officers break bad news to patients and relatives while still a student.'

While our students were facing these pressures, others were building up. Medical litigation was increasing sharply, and the number of court cases had more than doubled. There were fears that British medicine would soon become a medico-legal minefield, with lawyers encouraging patients to sue for negligence and doctors forced to practise expensive, conservative medicine calculated to protect their position in the event of a lawsuit.

Meanwhile, the organisation of health care was changing fast. Depending on the politicians and newspapers one paid heed to, the NHS was either undergoing a much-needed overhaul or experiencing a life-threatening crisis. Most doctors seemed to take the latter view, and fought a bitter campaign against a government determined to push through radical reforms that affected both hospital doctors and general practitioners. Morale declined sharply during the late 1980s and early 1990s. Central London was particularly badly affected because of the redistribution of NHS funds away from the teaching hospitals and towards the regions, and debates raged in the press about the future of London's medical schools.

One of the effects of the health service reforms was to turn patients into customers, and to apply 'market forces' to the health service, perhaps to the detriment of doctors' status in society. The old-style doctor-patient relationship, in which the patient placed his trust in the doctor, tacitly acknowledging his expertise and accepting his diagnosis and recommendations without question, was already strained by press reports of medical incompetence. Now the idea that a patient might 'shop around' for medical care threatened to destroy the unique role of the doctor as wise, disinterested, uniquely knowledgeable and more or less infallible.

With morale declining and the future uncertain, low pay and long hours could become insupportable. Our house officers observed school friends now working as solicitors or stockbrokers who had been earning high salaries for three or four years, and were now buying houses. All their non-medical friends had a better quality of life: they could take a modest social life, or even an unbroken night's sleep for granted.

It seems that Britain's sixth formers are coming to believe that all is not well in the world of medicine. Applications to medical schools have fallen steadily over the past fourteen years. In 1977 there were 12 098 applicants. By 1988 the figure had dropped to 9455. Many senior figures in medical education are predicting a crisis in their field. They fear that, unless the system is changed, bright A level students will spurn medicine and the quality of our doctors will decline.

One often-suggested improvement would be to reform the working patterns of junior hospital doctors by abolishing the current system which expects young professionals to do a full day's work and then stand by to work all night if necessary, without any time off the following day. British hospital doctors could work shifts, like their counterparts in Canada and Scandinavia. Critics of such a system insist that it would destroy the precious personal relationship which a house officer forms with his or her patients and would be detrimental to continuity of care.

Advocates of change, however, ask whether patients would prefer to be treated by someone who has been awake for the best part of seventy-two hours, and is rendered semi-competent by sleep deprivation, or by a fresh, alert, observant doctor who has read their notes, been well-briefed by colleagues and is on top of the job? Nurses, who are generally much closer to patients, have worked such a system for years, thanks to an efficient hand-over period between shifts. Some say the vested interest of senior hospital doctors militates against change: if shiftworking were introduced, there would be too few junior doctors to man the wards and *everyone* on the firm would have to do their share of active on-call duty, including registrars and consultants. Such a revolution would attract little support among consultants who themselves laboured for twenty years to escape the stranglehold of on-call commitments and who now often fill their spare time with lucrative private work.

Peter Richards was keenly aware that the system needed changing. He could still recall the arduousness of his first hospital jobs. 'It is the hardest time in one's whole professional career. I remember to this day the moment when I left my second house job and walked down the street without my bleep after a year incarcerated in the hospital. Since then, everything has got steadily better – at least as far as the physical demands of the job are concerned.' The Dean believed that conditions could be improved if students qualified sooner, but spent *two* years as house officers. If the number of staff in the grade was doubled, the on-call burden would be halved, and the presence of experienced second-year house officers would considerably help the new intake during their first few weeks. 'It would not cost a very great deal of money,' he commented. 'And, if it converted purgatory into a worthwhile educational experience, and a dissatisfied and miserable workforce into a happy one, it would be very worthwhile.'

Reform *is* needed, urgently. In a recent study of junior doctors' hours, commissioned by the Department of Health, a house officer in a teaching hospital who had just finished a typical week consisting of 121 hours on duty, 98 of them actually working, was quoted as follows:

'In years to come, people will be as shocked by the hours we work as by young boys being sent up chimneys a century ago. Eventually doctors must work a shift system, like everybody else.'

FURTHER READING

Learning Medicine, Peter Richards, British Medical Association, 1991.
A regularly updated paperback guide to medical education which explains how to get into medical school and paints a picture of life as a medical student.

Living Medicine, Peter Richards, Cambridge University Press, 1990.
The companion volume to **Learning Medicine**, which describes the final stages of medical school education and provides the information graduates need to plan their careers in medicine.

Invitation to Medicine, Douglas Black, Blackwell, 1987.
Designed to help those contemplating a career in medicine. Provides an overview of current medical knowledge and practice.

Doctors, Jonathan Gathorne-Hardy, Corgi, 1987.
Detailed interviews with fifty British GPs provide a wide-ranging picture of the life and work of family doctors today.

Doctors and Their Careers, Isobel Allen, Policy Studies Institute, 1988.
Report on a major survey of the views and experience of 600 male and female doctors who qualified in 1966, 1976 and 1981.

Any Room at the Top? A study of doctors and their careers, Isobel Allen, Policy Studies Institute, 1988.
A much shorter, paperback version of the above report. Reveals widespread anxiety about hours, pay, career structures and disillusionment with medicine.

Junior Doctors' Hours, Robin Dowie, Report for the DHSS published by the British Postgraduate Medical Federation, 1989.
A survey of the hours worked by 552 junior doctors. Grim reading.

The History of St Mary's Hospital Medical School, Sir Zachary Cope, Heinemann, 1954.
The official history of St Mary's.

APPLYING TO MEDICAL SCHOOLS

The Universities Central Council on Admissions (UCCA) publishes **How to Apply for Admission to a University**, an essential handbook for would-be students which explains when and how to apply to medical school and is revised annually. It is available from UCCA, PO Box 28, Cheltenham, Glos. GL50 1HY.

University Entrance: The Official Guide 1992, London: the Association of Commonwealth Universities. Contains a list of entry requirements including grades at A level for all university courses including medicine. It is updated annually.

The St Mary's Hospital Medical School prospectus, which is published annually, gives full details of the course at St Mary's and the organisation of the medical school. It is available from the Admissions Secretary, St Mary's Hospital Medical School, London W2 1PG.

INDEX